Protect Your KIDNEYS

A Doctor's Practical Guide to Kidney Health & Prevention

Dr Prabhat Das

MD, PhD, FACP

Better Health with Dr Das Series

Hardcover ISBN: 978-1-971672-52-6

Paperback ISBN: 978-1-971672-51-9

eBook ISBN: 978-1-971672-50-2

Printed in the United States of America

Disclaimer

This book is intended solely for educational and informational purposes. It is not meant to replace personal medical advice, diagnosis, or treatment.

Although I am a licensed physician, reading this book does not establish a doctor-patient relationship. Each individual's health condition, medical history, and risk factors are unique. Any medical decision should be made in partnership with your own healthcare professional who understands your specific situation.

Medical science is continually advancing. New research and updated guidelines may lead to changes in recommendations over time.

About the Author

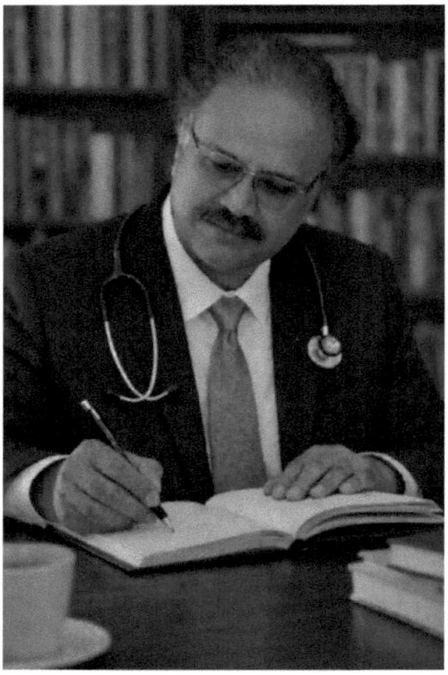

I am Dr Prabhat Das, MD, PhD, FACP. My journey in medicine began in India and, over the past thirty-five years, has continued in the United States, where I have had the privilege of caring for patients across a wide range of medical settings. I am trained in Internal Medicine, Pulmonary Diseases, and Critical Care. For me, medicine has never been just a profession. It has been a lifelong commitment shaped by learning, service, and a deep respect for the trust patients place in their physician.

Over the years, I have had the honor of caring for patients in many different situations. I have seen individuals in my office for routine concerns, treated urgent conditions in busy emergency rooms, managed serious illnesses in the hospital, and cared for critically ill patients in intensive care units. Each setting has taught me something valuable. Each patient has added to my understanding of what it truly means to care for another human being.

But one lesson has stood above all others. Medicine is not only about tests, diagnoses, or treatments. It is about people. It is about listening carefully, understanding fears that are often left unspoken, and guiding patients through uncertainty with clarity and compassion. Again and again, I have seen that what people want most is simple, trustworthy information. They want to understand what is happening in their bodies. They want to feel confident about the decisions they are making for their health and for their families.

These experiences have deeply shaped how I think about health, illness, prevention, and the human side of healing.

That is the reason behind the '**Better Health with Dr Das Series'**. Through these books, I hope to reach individuals I may never meet in person but who are searching for clear and reliable guidance. In today's world, health information is everywhere, yet much of it is confusing, overwhelming, and sometimes misleading. My goal is to cut through that noise and present important medical topics in a way that is simple, practical, and reassuring.

Every page of this series is guided by two foundations: reliable scientific knowledge and decades of real-world clinical experience. I want you, the reader, to feel informed, confident, and empowered. Not overwhelmed. Not confused. But clear about what you can do, step by step, to improve your health.

If even one reader feels less anxious, more informed, or better prepared to take control of their health after reading these books, then this work has served its purpose.

Helping people live healthier, longer, more confident and better-informed lives remains one of the greatest privileges of my life.

Table of Contents:

CHAPTER 1: Why Kidney Health Deserves Your Attention

The Quiet Organs Most People Never Think About

Most people do not spend much time thinking about their kidneys.

That is understandable. You cannot see them. You do not feel them working. They do their job silently, faithfully, and without asking for attention. Day after day, year after year, they continue their work in the background while life moves on.

But that quiet work is essential.

Your kidneys are among the most important organs in your body. They remove waste from the blood, help balance fluids, regulate important minerals, support healthy blood pressure, and play a role in keeping your bones and blood healthy. They are not simply organs that make urine. They are part of the body's internal control system, constantly helping maintain order and stability.

When they are healthy, you usually do not notice them at all. That is a sign of how well they are doing their job.

The problem is that when kidney trouble begins, it often starts just as quietly.

Why Kidney Problems Are So Easy to Miss

One of the most important things I want the reader to understand from the very beginning is this:

Early kidney disease often does not cause pain or obvious symptoms.

That is what makes it so deceptive.

A person may feel well, go to work, enjoy family life, sleep normally, and carry on with daily routines, while early kidney damage is already developing. There may be no dramatic warning sign. No strong signal from the body saying that something is wrong. In many cases, the first clue comes from a routine blood test or urine test.

This surprises many people.

I have seen patients look genuinely shocked when they are told that their kidney function is not normal. Their response is often very natural: "But doctor, I feel fine."

That reaction makes perfect sense. In most situations, we expect illness to announce itself. We expect pain, weakness, or some obvious change. Kidney disease often does not behave that way in the beginning.

That is why awareness matters so much.

The Kidneys Do Much More Than Most People Realize

Many people think of the kidneys in a very limited way. They assume the kidneys simply filter blood and produce urine.

They do much more than that.

Healthy kidneys help:

- remove waste products from the body
- control the right amount of water in the body
- balance minerals such as sodium and potassium
- support healthy blood pressure
- help maintain bone health
- contribute to red blood cell production

This means kidney health affects far more than urination. It influences energy, circulation, swelling, blood pressure, bone strength, and overall well-being.

When kidney function begins to decline, the effects do not stay confined to one corner of the body. Over time, the entire body feels the consequences.

That is why kidney health deserves more respect than it usually gets.

Why This Topic Matters More Than Ever

Kidney disease is not a rare problem affecting only a small number of people. It is common, especially in adults over forty and in people who already live with diabetes, high blood pressure, heart disease, obesity, or recurrent kidney stones.

Many people are walking around with early kidney disease and do not know it.

That is not because they are careless. It is because the condition often remains silent until it becomes more advanced.

This silence creates danger, but it also creates an opportunity.

If kidney problems are found early, there is often a great deal we can do. We can control the risk factors more carefully. We can adjust medications. We can improve diet and lifestyle. We can monitor progress closely. In many cases, we can slow the disease and reduce complications.

That is the encouraging side of this story.

This is not a book meant to frighten the reader. It is a book meant to help the reader recognize a problem early enough to do something meaningful about it.

Who Should Be Especially Careful

Although everyone should have some basic awareness of kidney health, some people need to be particularly alert.

You should pay close attention to your kidneys if you have:

- diabetes
- high blood pressure
- heart disease
- a family history of kidney disease
- recurrent kidney stones
- regular use of certain pain medicines
- increasing age, especially after midlife

These are common situations. That is exactly why this subject is so important.

A person may think, “My sugar is only mildly high,” or “My blood pressure is not that bad,” or “I only take pain medicine once in a while.” But many health problems do their damage quietly over time. What seems mild today may become significant after years of neglect.

The kidneys often pay that price.

A Common Story From Everyday Practice

Let me put this into a real-life setting.

A middle-aged man comes in for a routine visit. He is busy, active, and not particularly worried about his health. He has had high blood pressure for several years, but because he has no major symptoms, he has not taken it very seriously. He sleeps reasonably well. He works every day. He has no pain. Nothing dramatic has happened.

Routine blood work is done.

His creatinine is mildly elevated. His kidney function is lower than expected. His urine test shows early signs of damage.

Now, for the first time, the kidneys become part of the conversation.

He is surprised. Sometimes patients are not just surprised, they are unsettled. They feel that their body has kept a secret from them. They ask how this can happen when they have been feeling normal.

The answer is simple, but important:

Kidney disease often begins in silence.

This is exactly why regular testing matters. It gives us a chance to discover a problem before the body is forced to reveal it in a harder way.

Why Early Detection Changes the Future

This point cannot be overstated.

When kidney disease is found early, the future can be very different.

At an early stage, there is time to act. Blood pressure can be controlled more carefully. Blood sugar can be improved. Harmful medicines can be reduced or avoided. Diet can be adjusted. Weight can be managed. Stones and infections can be evaluated before they cause more harm. Follow-up can be planned in a thoughtful way rather than in a rushed and frightened way.

Early detection gives people something precious in medicine: time.

And in kidney disease, time matters.

The earlier a person understands what is happening, the greater the chance of slowing the process and protecting long-term health.

The Real Purpose of This Book

This book is not meant to overwhelm the reader with complicated medical language. It is meant to make an important subject clear, practical, and useful.

I want the reader to come away with three things.

First, a clear understanding of what the kidneys do and why they matter.

Second, a practical understanding of how kidney disease begins, how it is found, and what can be done about it.

Third, a sense of hope and control.

Too many people hear the word "kidney" and immediately think of fear, dialysis, or helplessness. That is not the whole story. In fact, for many people, the more relevant story is prevention, early diagnosis, careful management, and long-term protection.

That is the story this book aims to tell.

Doctor's Pearl

Do not wait for your kidneys to complain before you pay attention to them.

Common Mistake to Avoid

Assuming that feeling well means your kidneys must be healthy.

Red Flag Warning

If you have diabetes, high blood pressure, swelling, changes in urination, blood in urine, or a family history of kidney disease, do not delay proper evaluation.

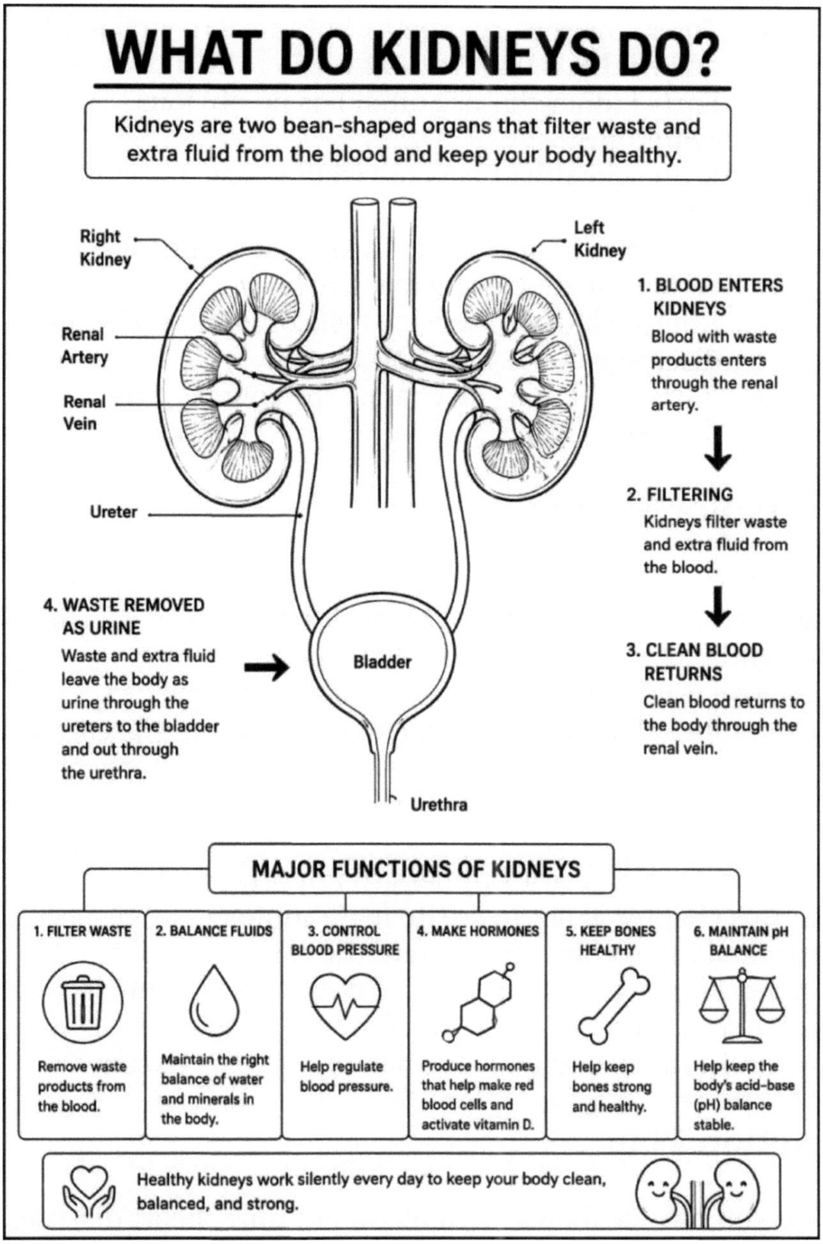
WHAT DO KIDNEYS DO?
Kidneys are two bean-shaped organs that filter waste and extra fluid from the blood and keep your body healthy.
Right Kidney
Left Kidney
Renal Artery
Renal Vein
Ureter
Bladder
Urethra
1. BLOOD ENTERS KIDNEYS
Blood with waste products enters through the renal artery.
2. FILTERING
Kidneys filter waste and extra fluid from the blood.
3. CLEAN BLOOD RETURNS
Clean blood returns to the body through the renal vein.
4. WASTE REMOVED AS URINE
Waste and extra fluid leave the body as urine through the ureters to the bladder and out through the urethra.
MAJOR FUNCTIONS OF KIDNEYS
1. FILTER WASTE
Remove waste products from the blood.
2. BALANCE FLUIDS
Maintain the right balance of water and minerals in the body.
3. CONTROL BLOOD PRESSURE
Help regulate blood pressure.
4. MAKE HORMONES
Produce hormones that help make red blood cells and activate vitamin D.
5. KEEP BONES HEALTHY
Help keep bones strong and healthy.
6. MAINTAIN pH BALANCE
Help keep the body's acid-base (pH) balance stable.
Healthy kidneys work silently every day to keep your body clean, balanced, and strong.

Key Points

- The kidneys work quietly, but they are vital to life and health.
- Early kidney disease often has no obvious symptoms.
- Kidney health affects the whole body, not just urination.
- Diabetes, high blood pressure, age, stones, and certain medicines increase risk.
- Routine blood and urine tests often detect kidney disease before symptoms appear.
- Early detection can change the course of the disease.

Chapter Summary

Most people do not think much about their kidneys until something goes wrong. Yet these quiet organs perform essential work every day, helping maintain balance, remove waste, support blood pressure, and protect overall health. The great challenge with kidney disease is that it often begins silently. A person may feel perfectly well while early damage is already present.

That is what makes awareness so important. The purpose of this chapter is not to create fear, but to create respect for the kidneys and attention to the early signs of trouble. When kidney problems are discovered early, there is often a meaningful chance to slow progression, reduce complications, and preserve health for years to come.

Action Plan

• If you have diabetes, high blood pressure, heart disease, or a family history of kidney disease, make sure kidney testing becomes part of your routine care.

• Do not ignore simple blood and urine tests. They often reveal problems long before symptoms appear.

• Review your risk factors honestly, especially blood pressure, blood sugar, weight, pain medicine use, and any history of stones.

• Begin thinking of kidney health as part of your overall long-term health, not as a separate issue.

• Read the rest of this book with one clear goal: early awareness, early action, and better protection for the future.

Transition to the Next Chapter

Now that we have started with the quiet importance of the kidneys, the next question is a natural one: how do kidney problems actually begin? In the next chapter, we will look at how damage develops, why it often progresses slowly, and why the earliest changes are so easy to miss.

CHAPTER 2: How Kidney Problems Begin and Progress Quietly

A System Built for Balance

In a healthy body, the kidneys work with remarkable precision.

They filter blood continuously, remove waste, and adjust fluid and mineral balance with quiet accuracy. If you drink more water, they remove the excess. If you lose fluid through heat or illness, they conserve what the body needs. If minerals shift, they correct the imbalance.

This fine control goes on every moment of your life, without your awareness.

For years, even decades, this system works smoothly. That is why most people assume it will always remain that way.

But like any system under constant demand, it can begin to weaken when exposed to long-term stress.

---

ow Damage Usually Starts

---

idney disease rarely begins with a dramatic event.

In most people, it starts slowly.

At first:

- There is mild stress on the kidneys
- The kidneys compensate
- You feel completely normal

Then, over time:

- Filtering becomes less efficient
- Small changes appear in blood or urine tests
- The kidneys begin to lose their reserve

This early stage is easy to miss.

There is no pain. No clear warning. Life continues as usual.

Yet this is the stage where action matters most.

The Two Main Patterns: Sudden and Slow

It helps to understand that kidney problems usually follow one of two patterns.

Acute Kidney Injury

This is a sudden drop in kidney function over hours or days.

It may be triggered by:

- Dehydration
- Severe illness
- Certain medications
- Blockage of urine flow

The important point is that this type of injury is often reversible if treated promptly.

Chronic Kidney Disease

This develops slowly over months or years.

It is usually related to:

- Diabetes
- High blood pressure
- Long-term stress on the kidneys

This form may not be fully reversible, but it can often be slowed significantly.

Understanding the difference between these two patterns helps guide treatment and expectations.

The Most Common Causes in Daily Practice

In real life, a few conditions account for most kidney problems.

Diabetes
Persistently high blood sugar gradually damages the tiny filters in the kidneys.

High Blood Pressure
Constant pressure injures the delicate blood vessels inside the kidneys.

Medications and Toxins
Frequent or improper use of certain drugs can reduce blood flow or directly harm kidney tissue.

Obstruction
Anything that blocks urine flow, such as stones or prostate enlargement, can damage the kidneys over time.

Infections and Inflammation
Repeated infections or immune-related conditions can slowly affect kidney structure.

Often, more than one of these factors is present.

The Role of Aging and Lifestyle

As we age, kidney function naturally declines to some extent.

But the rate of decline varies widely.

Lifestyle plays a major role.

Factors that speed up damage include:

- Poor control of blood sugar
- Uncontrolled blood pressure
- High salt intake
- Excess weight
- Smoking
- Lack of physical activity

On the other hand, simple healthy habits can slow the process and preserve kidney function for many years.

Why You Do Not Feel It Early

This is one of the most important ideas in this book.

The kidneys have a large reserve capacity.

Even if part of their function is lost, the remaining part continues to work well enough to maintain balance.

This is helpful, but it also creates a problem.

Because:

- There is no pain
- There is no clear signal
- Daily life feels unchanged

The disease can progress quietly.

By the time symptoms appear, a significant amount of function may already be lost.

A Common Clinical Situation

A patient with long-standing diabetes comes for routine follow-up.

He feels fine. There are no kidney-related complaints.

Tests show:

- Small amounts of protein in urine

- A slight reduction in kidney function

This is the beginning of kidney damage.

At this stage:

- Nothing feels wrong
- But something important has started

With proper care, the process can often be slowed.

If ignored, it may continue silently.

Two Possible Paths

At this point, the journey can take two very different directions.

In one path:

- The problem is recognized early
- Risk factors are controlled
- Follow-up is regular
- Kidney function remains stable for years

In the other:

- Early signs are ignored
- Risk factors remain uncontrolled
- Monitoring is irregular
- The disease progresses

The difference is not chance.

It is awareness and action.

Doctor's Pearl

Kidney damage often begins long before you feel anything. Early action makes the greatest difference.

Common Mistake to Avoid

Waiting for symptoms before taking kidney health seriously.

Red Flag Warning

Be especially cautious if you have:

- Long-standing diabetes
- Poorly controlled blood pressure
- Frequent use of pain medications
- Recurrent kidney stones

These increase the risk of kidney damage.

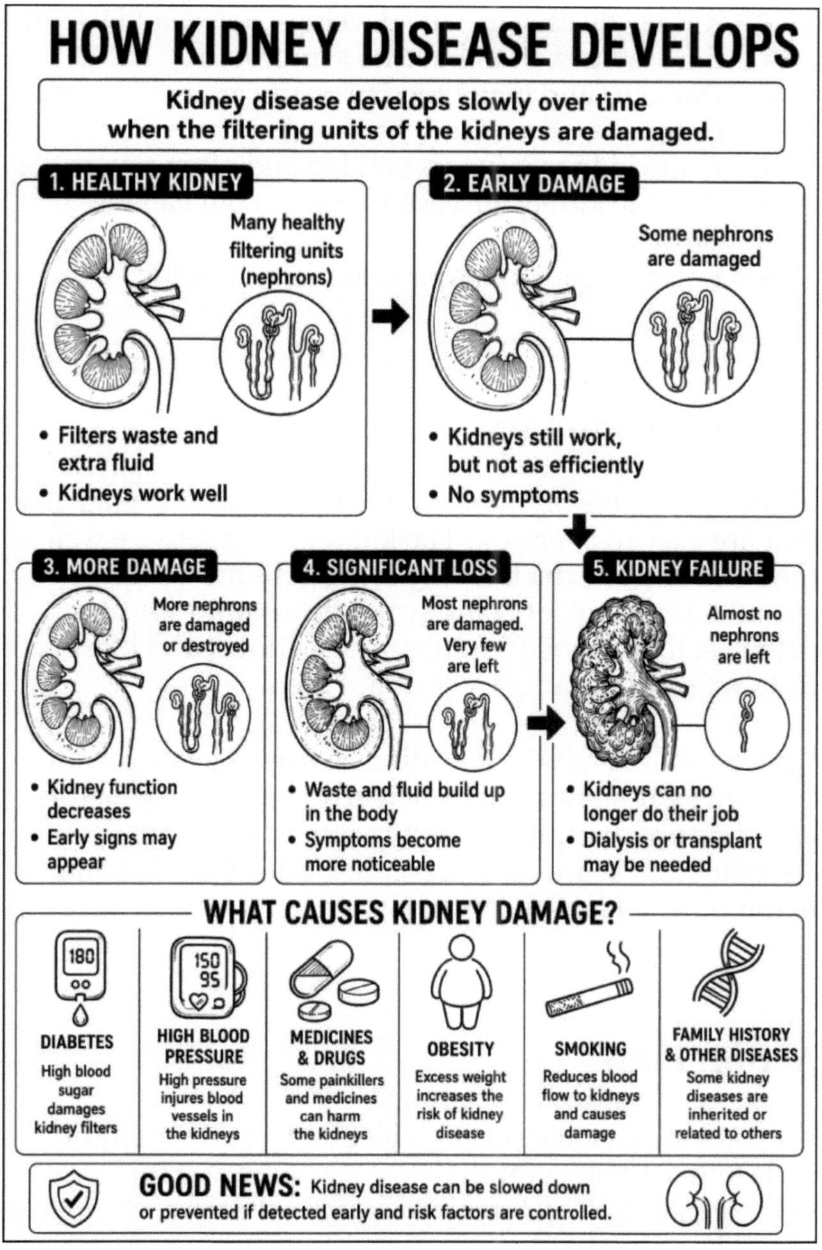
HOW KIDNEY DISEASE DEVELOPS
Kidney disease develops slowly over time when the filtering units of the kidneys are damaged.
1. HEALTHY KIDNEY
Many healthy filtering units (nephrons)
• Filters waste and extra fluid
• Kidneys work well
2. EARLY DAMAGE
Some nephrons are damaged
• Kidneys still work, but not as efficiently
• No symptoms
3. MORE DAMAGE
More nephrons are damaged or destroyed
• Kidney function decreases
• Early signs may appear
4. SIGNIFICANT LOSS
Most nephrons are damaged. Very few are left
• Waste and fluid build up in the body
• Symptoms become more noticeable
5. KIDNEY FAILURE
Almost no nephrons are left
• Kidneys can no longer do their job
• Dialysis or transplant may be needed
WHAT CAUSES KIDNEY DAMAGE?
180
DIABETES
High blood sugar damages kidney filters
150
95
HIGH BLOOD PRESSURE
High pressure injures blood vessels in the kidneys
MEDICINES & DRUGS
Some painkillers and medicines can harm the kidneys
OBESITY
Excess weight increases the risk of kidney disease
SMOKING
Reduces blood flow to kidneys and causes damage
FAMILY HISTORY & OTHER DISEASES
Some kidney diseases are inherited or related to others
GOOD NEWS: Kidney disease can be slowed down or prevented if detected early and risk factors are controlled.

Key Points

- Kidney disease usually develops slowly and silently
- Early stages often have no symptoms
- Diabetes and high blood pressure are the leading causes
- Acute kidney injury is sudden and often reversible
- Chronic kidney disease is gradual but can be slowed
- Lifestyle plays a major role in progression

Chapter Summary

Kidney problems often begin quietly, with small changes that are easy to overlook. The kidneys compensate well in the early stages, which is why symptoms are usually absent. Over time, ongoing stress from conditions such as diabetes, high blood pressure, medications, and lifestyle factors leads to gradual loss of function.

Understanding how kidney disease begins gives you an advantage. It allows you to act early, control risk factors, and slow progression. In many cases, simple and consistent measures can preserve kidney function and maintain good health for years.

Action Plan

• If you have diabetes or high blood pressure, monitor and control them carefully
• Get regular kidney function tests as advised
• Avoid unnecessary or prolonged use of pain medications
• Maintain a healthy weight and stay active
• Reduce salt intake and follow a balanced diet

Transition to the Next Chapter

Now that you understand how kidney problems begin, the next step is to recognize the early warning signs. In the next chapter, we will look at the subtle symptoms and red flags that should never be ignored.

CHAPTER 3: Warning Signs You Should Never Ignore

When the Body Speaks Softly

Kidney disease has a quiet beginning. That is its most challenging feature.

In the early stages, the body often does not raise a clear alarm. There is no sharp pain, no dramatic symptom, nothing that forces you to stop and take notice. Life continues in its usual rhythm.

But if you pay close attention, the body does send signals. They are gentle, easy to dismiss, and often explained away as fatigue, age, or a busy routine.

Learning to recognize these early signs is one of the most valuable skills you can develop.

Subtle Changes That Deserve Attention

The first signs of kidney trouble are usually mild.

You may notice:

- A slight drop in your usual energy
- Feeling tired without a clear reason
- Mild swelling around the ankles by evening
- Puffiness around the eyes in the morning

Individually, these may not seem important. Together, they may be telling you that something needs to be checked.

The mistake many people make is to ignore these small changes until they become more obvious.

Urine: A Simple but Important Clue

If there is one place where kidney health often reveals itself early, it is in the urine.

Changes to watch for include:

- Foamy urine, which may suggest protein loss
- Blood in urine, appearing pink, red, or tea-colored
- Dark or unusually concentrated urine
- Passing urine more or less often than usual
- Waking up frequently at night to urinate

These changes do not always mean kidney disease, but they should never be ignored.

They deserve proper evaluation.

When Symptoms Become More Noticeable

As kidney function declines further, symptoms become easier to recognize.

At this stage, the body is no longer able to maintain balance as efficiently.

You may experience:

- Persistent fatigue
- Loss of appetite
- Nausea
- Difficulty concentrating
- A general sense of not feeling well

These symptoms develop gradually and are often attributed to other causes. That is why they are frequently overlooked.

Swelling and Fluid Retention

One of the clearer signs of kidney trouble is fluid retention.

When the kidneys cannot remove excess fluid effectively:

- Swelling appears in the feet and ankles
- The face may look puffy, especially in the morning
- Shoes or rings may feel tighter than usual

In more advanced situations:

- Fluid may affect breathing
- Shortness of breath may develop

This is a sign that needs prompt attention.

Blood Pressure: A Silent Indicator

Blood pressure and kidney health are closely connected.

Sometimes the first sign of kidney disease is:

- A rise in blood pressure
- Difficulty controlling blood pressure with usual treatment

Because high blood pressure itself often has no symptoms, this change may go unnoticed unless it is measured regularly.

When the Situation Becomes Urgent

While many symptoms develop slowly, some situations require immediate attention.

Do not delay if you notice:

- Visible blood in urine
- Severe or rapidly increasing swelling
- Very little or no urine
- Persistent vomiting
- Shortness of breath
- Confusion or unusual drowsiness

These signs may indicate serious complications that need urgent care.

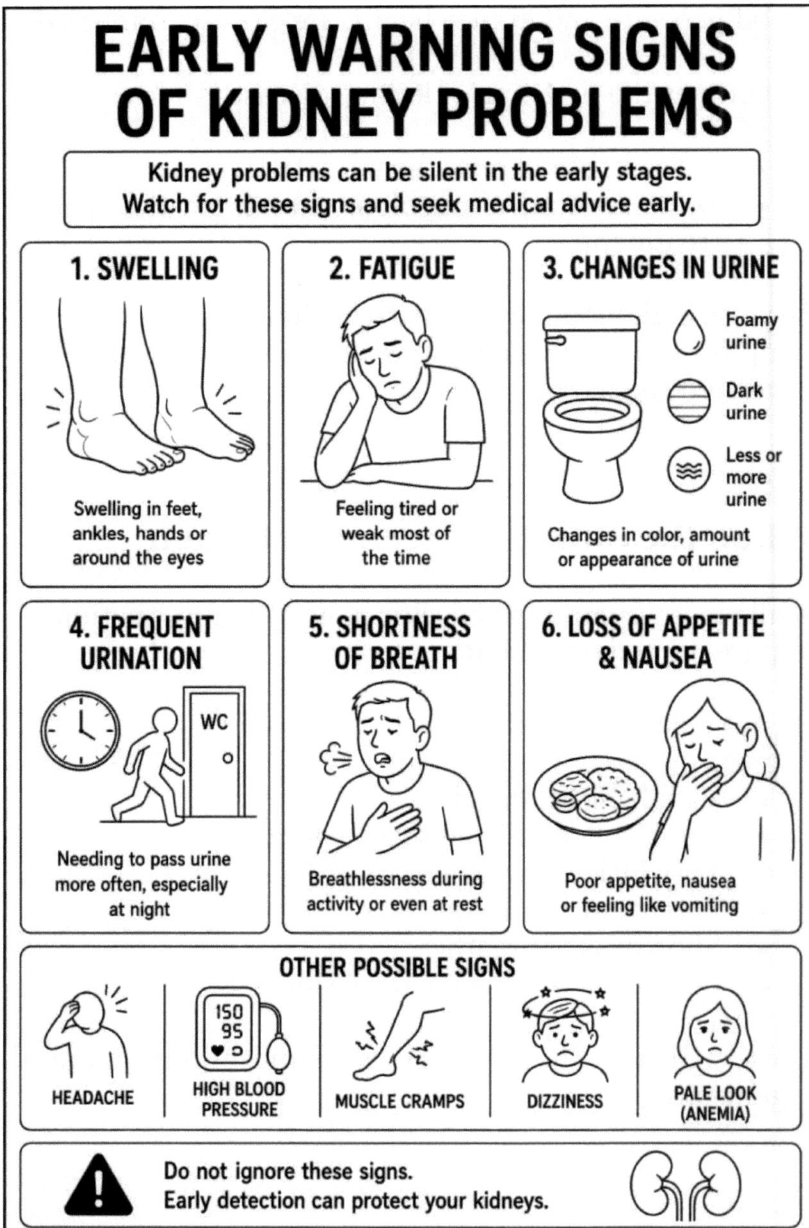
EARLY WARNING SIGNS OF KIDNEY PROBLEMS
Kidney problems can be silent in the early stages.
Watch for these signs and seek medical advice early.
1. SWELLING
Swelling in feet, ankles, hands or around the eyes
2. FATIGUE
Feeling tired or weak most of the time
3. CHANGES IN URINE
Foamy urine
Dark urine
Less or more urine
Changes in color, amount or appearance of urine
4. FREQUENT URINATION
WC
Needing to pass urine more often, especially at night
5. SHORTNESS OF BREATH
Breathlessness during activity or even at rest
6. LOSS OF APPETITE & NAUSEA
Poor appetite, nausea or feeling like vomiting
OTHER POSSIBLE SIGNS
HEADACHE
150
95
HIGH BLOOD PRESSURE
MUSCLE CRAMPS
DIZZINESS
PALE LOOK (ANEMIA)
Do not ignore these signs.
Early detection can protect your kidneys.

A Story You May Recognize

A patient with long-standing high blood pressure begins to feel slightly more tired than usual.

He notices mild swelling in his feet in the evening. He assumes it is due to long hours at work or getting older.

Months pass.

Eventually, tests reveal moderate kidney dysfunction.

Nothing dramatic happened. The body gave quiet signals, but they were ignored.

This is a common story, and it can be prevented.

Doctor's Pearl

In kidney disease, the early signs are often soft. Listening early makes all the difference.

Common Mistake to Avoid

Dismissing fatigue, swelling, or urine changes as minor or age-related without checking.

Red Flag Warning

Seek medical attention if you notice:

- Blood in urine
- Sudden swelling
- Reduced urine output
- Persistent nausea or vomiting
- Shortness of breath

Key Points

- Early kidney disease often has no obvious symptoms
- Subtle signs include fatigue, swelling, and urine changes
- Urine provides important early clues
- Symptoms become clearer as disease progresses
- Some signs require urgent medical care

Chapter Summary

Kidney disease often begins quietly, making it easy to miss in its early stages. However, the body does provide subtle signals such as mild fatigue, swelling, and changes in urination. As the condition progresses, symptoms become more noticeable and may affect overall well-being.

Recognizing these early signs and acting on them can lead to timely diagnosis and treatment. This can slow progression and prevent serious complications. Paying attention to your body is one of the simplest and most effective ways to protect your kidney health.

Action Plan

- Pay attention to any changes in your urine
- Monitor for swelling in the legs, feet, or around the eyes
- Check your blood pressure regularly
- Do not ignore persistent fatigue
- Seek medical advice if any unusual symptoms appear

Transition to the Next Chapter

Now that you know how kidney disease may show itself, the next step is to understand how it affects the rest of the body. In the next chapter, we will look at why kidney disease is not just a kidney problem, but a condition that influences overall health.

CHAPTER 4: How Kidney Disease Affects the Entire Body

It Is Not Just About the Kidneys

When people hear that their kidneys are not working well, they often assume the problem is limited to urine or fluid balance.

That is a very natural thought, but it is not correct.

The kidneys are deeply connected with almost every major system in the body. When their function begins to decline, the effects are felt far beyond the kidneys themselves.

Over time, kidney disease becomes a whole-body condition.

It influences the heart, blood, bones, brain, and overall energy. Understanding this changes the way you think about kidney disease. It is not something small or isolated. It is something that deserves careful attention.

The Heart and Kidneys Work Together

The heart and kidneys share a close and constant relationship.

The kidneys help control fluid levels and blood pressure. The heart depends on this balance to function efficiently.

When kidney function declines:

- Fluid may build up in the body
- Blood pressure may rise
- The heart has to work harder

Over time, this increases the risk of:

- Heart attack
- Stroke
- Heart failure

In fact, many patients with kidney disease face heart-related problems even before kidney failure becomes severe.

Protecting the kidneys also protects the heart.

Effects on Blood: Why Fatigue Develops

Healthy kidneys produce a hormone that helps the body make red blood cells.

When kidney function declines:

- This hormone is reduced
- Red blood cell production falls
- Anemia develops

This leads to:

- Persistent fatigue
- Low energy
- Reduced stamina

Patients often feel tired without understanding why. It is not just weakness. It reflects a deeper imbalance in the body.

Bones and Minerals: A Delicate System

The kidneys help maintain the balance of calcium, phosphorus, and vitamin D.

These are essential for healthy bones.

When kidney function is reduced:

- Calcium balance is disturbed
- Phosphorus levels may rise
- Vitamin D activation decreases

Over time, this can lead to:

- Weak bones
- Bone pain
- Increased risk of fractures

This problem develops slowly and is often overlooked until it becomes significant.

Brain and Mental Clarity

As kidney disease progresses, waste products begin to accumulate in the blood.

These can affect the brain.

You may notice:

- Difficulty concentrating
- Memory changes
- Poor sleep
- Irritability

In more advanced stages:

- Confusion may develop

These changes can affect daily life in subtle but important ways.

Fluid Retention and Swelling

One of the more visible effects of kidney disease is fluid retention.

When the kidneys cannot remove excess fluid:

- Swelling appears in the legs and ankles
- Puffiness develops around the eyes
- Body weight may increase

In more serious cases:

- Fluid can affect the lungs
- Breathing becomes difficult

This is a sign that needs prompt attention.

Muscles and Energy

Electrolyte imbalance and waste buildup affect muscles.

Patients may experience:

- Muscle cramps
- Weakness
- Reduced endurance

Combined with anemia, this leads to the overall fatigue that many patients describe.

It is usually not one single cause, but a combination of factors.

Hormonal and Internal Balance

The kidneys play a role in several important hormonal systems.

When kidney function declines:

- Blood pressure regulation is affected
- Red blood cell production decreases
- Bone metabolism changes

At the same time, waste products accumulate, leading to:

- Loss of appetite

- Nausea
- General discomfort

These changes may seem unrelated at first, but they are all connected.

A Clinical Picture That Brings It Together

Consider a patient with long-standing kidney disease.

Over time, he notices:

- Increasing fatigue
- Swelling in the legs
- Shortness of breath with activity
- Difficulty controlling blood pressure

At first, these may seem like separate problems.

In reality, they are all part of the same process.

The kidneys are no longer able to maintain balance, and the whole body is affected.

Doctor's Pearl

Kidney disease is not just a kidney problem. It is a whole-body condition.

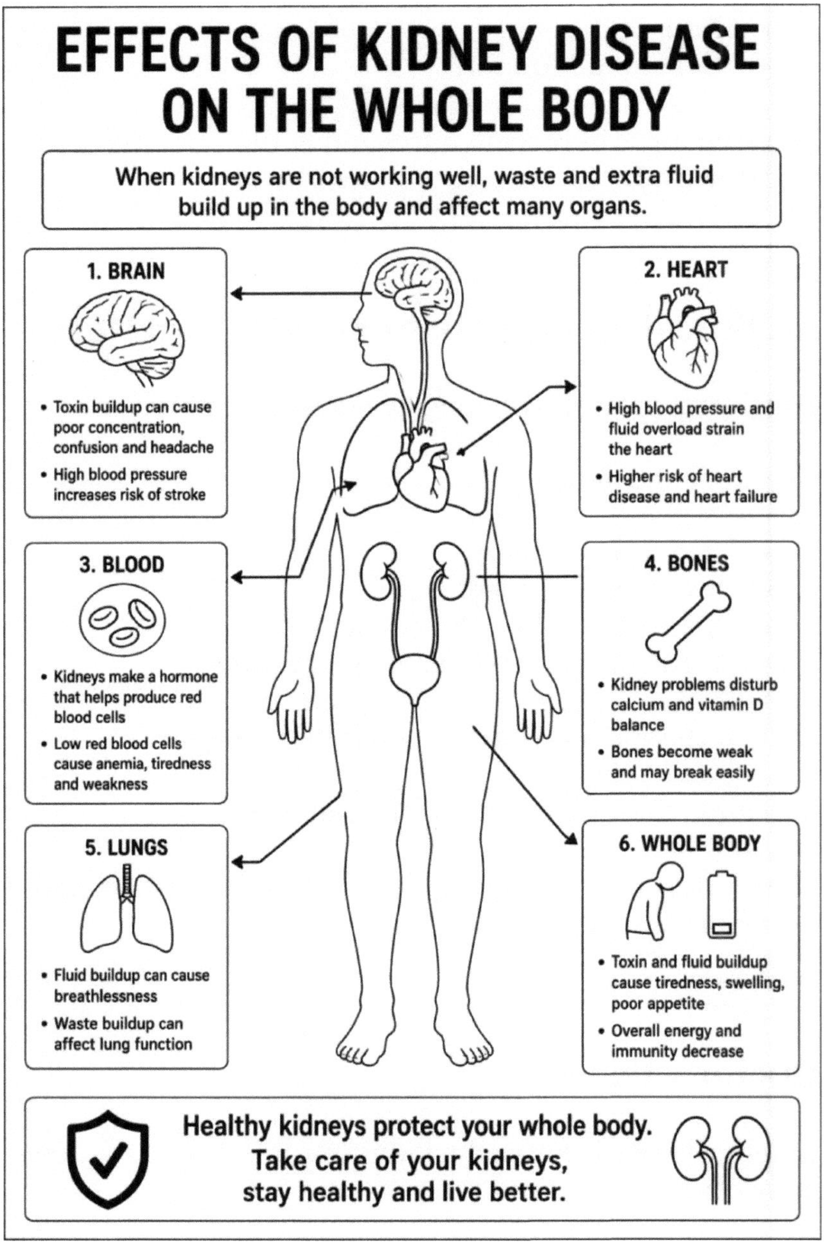
EFFECTS OF KIDNEY DISEASE ON THE WHOLE BODY
When kidneys are not working well, waste and extra fluid build up in the body and affect many organs.
1. BRAIN
• Toxin buildup can cause poor concentration, confusion and headache
• High blood pressure increases risk of stroke
2. HEART
• High blood pressure and fluid overload strain the heart
• Higher risk of heart disease and heart failure
3. BLOOD
• Kidneys make a hormone that helps produce red blood cells
• Low red blood cells cause anemia, tiredness and weakness
4. BONES
• Kidney problems disturb calcium and vitamin D balance
• Bones become weak and may break easily
5. LUNGS
• Fluid buildup can cause breathlessness
• Waste buildup can affect lung function
6. WHOLE BODY
• Toxin and fluid buildup cause tiredness, swelling, poor appetite
• Overall energy and immunity decrease
Healthy kidneys protect your whole body.
Take care of your kidneys,
stay healthy and live better.

Common Mistake to Avoid

Thinking that kidney disease only affects urine and nothing else.

Red Flag Warning

Seek urgent medical attention if you notice:

- Sudden shortness of breath
- Rapid swelling
- Confusion
- Chest discomfort

Key Points

- Kidney disease affects multiple organ systems
- It increases the risk of heart disease
- It can cause anemia and fatigue
- It weakens bones over time
- It affects mental clarity and sleep
- Fluid imbalance can lead to swelling and breathing problems

---

Chapter Summary

Kidney disease affects far more than the kidneys. It influences the heart, blood, bones, brain, and overall energy. These effects develop gradually but can significantly impact quality of life.

Understanding this broader impact helps you recognize why early detection and proper management are so important. Treating kidney disease is not only about preserving kidney function. It is about protecting the entire body.

Action Plan

- Monitor your blood pressure regularly
- Pay attention to fatigue, swelling, or breathing changes
- Keep regular follow-up appointments
- Follow dietary and medical advice
- Report any new or worsening symptoms early

Transition to the Next Chapter

Now that you understand how kidney disease affects the body, the next step is to look at what happens when it is not properly managed. In the next chapter, we will discuss the complications that can develop and why timely care makes such a difference.

CHAPTER 5: The Consequences of Delay: What Happens When Kidney Disease Is Ignored

When a Quiet Problem Becomes a Serious One

Kidney disease rarely starts with a crisis.

It begins quietly, often with small changes in blood or urine tests. At that stage, many people feel well and carry on with daily life. Because there are no clear symptoms, the problem is easy to ignore.

But kidney disease does not remain quiet forever.

If it is not recognized and managed in time, the effects slowly build. What started as a mild abnormality can gradually turn into a complex condition affecting multiple systems in the body.

This is not a sudden transformation. It is a slow progression that becomes more difficult to control with time.

The Gradual Loss of Kidney Function

The most direct consequence of untreated kidney disease is a steady decline in kidney function.

In the beginning:

- The kidneys compensate
- Changes in lab values are mild

As time passes:

- Filtering capacity decreases
- Waste products begin to accumulate
- The body struggles to maintain balance

If this process continues unchecked, it can eventually lead to kidney failure, where the kidneys can no longer support the body on their own.

At that stage, dialysis or transplantation may be required.

The Heart Often Suffers First

One of the most important complications of kidney disease involves the heart.

When the kidneys are not working properly:

- Blood pressure tends to rise
- Fluid may accumulate
- Blood vessels are affected

This places extra strain on the heart.

As a result, the risk of:

- Heart attack
- Stroke

- Heart failure

increases significantly.

In many cases, patients with kidney disease are more likely to face heart problems than kidney failure itself.

Fluid Overload and Breathing Problems

Healthy kidneys maintain the right amount of fluid in the body.

When this function is impaired:

- Fluid begins to build up
- Swelling develops in the legs and ankles
- Weight increases gradually

In more advanced stages:

- Fluid can accumulate in the lungs
- Breathing becomes difficult

This is not just uncomfortable. It can become a medical emergency if not treated promptly.

Electrolyte Imbalance: A Hidden Risk

The kidneys help maintain a careful balance of minerals.

When this balance is disturbed:

- Potassium levels may rise
- Sodium levels may change
- Acid levels may increase

High potassium levels are particularly dangerous because they can affect the heart's rhythm.

These imbalances may not always cause clear symptoms at first, which is why regular monitoring is essential.

Anemia and Persistent Fatigue

As kidney function declines, the body produces fewer red blood cells.

This leads to anemia.

Patients often experience:

- Ongoing fatigue
- Reduced stamina
- Shortness of breath with activity

This is one of the most common and frustrating symptoms in later stages.

Bone Weakness and Mineral Disorders

Kidney disease disrupts the balance of calcium, phosphorus, and vitamin D.

Over time, this can result in:

- Weak bones
- Bone pain
- Increased risk of fractures

This complication develops gradually and is often not recognized until it becomes significant.

Loss of Appetite and General Decline

As waste products build up in the body, they affect appetite and digestion.

Patients may notice:

- Reduced appetite
- Nausea
- Weight loss
- General weakness

These changes contribute to a decline in overall health.

When the Condition Becomes Critical

In advanced stages, the body can no longer compensate.

At this point:

- Waste products reach high levels
- Fluid overload becomes severe
- Electrolyte balance becomes unstable

This stage requires urgent medical care and often leads to the need for dialysis or transplantation.

A Common Clinical Pattern

A patient with diabetes and high blood pressure has mild kidney abnormalities for several years.

Because he feels well, follow-up is irregular.

Gradually:

- Kidney function declines
- Swelling develops
- Blood pressure becomes difficult to control
- Fatigue increases

Eventually, he presents with severe symptoms.

This pattern is not rare.

In many cases, early action could have slowed or prevented this progression.

Doctor's Pearl

Most complications of kidney disease can be delayed or prevented with early and consistent care.

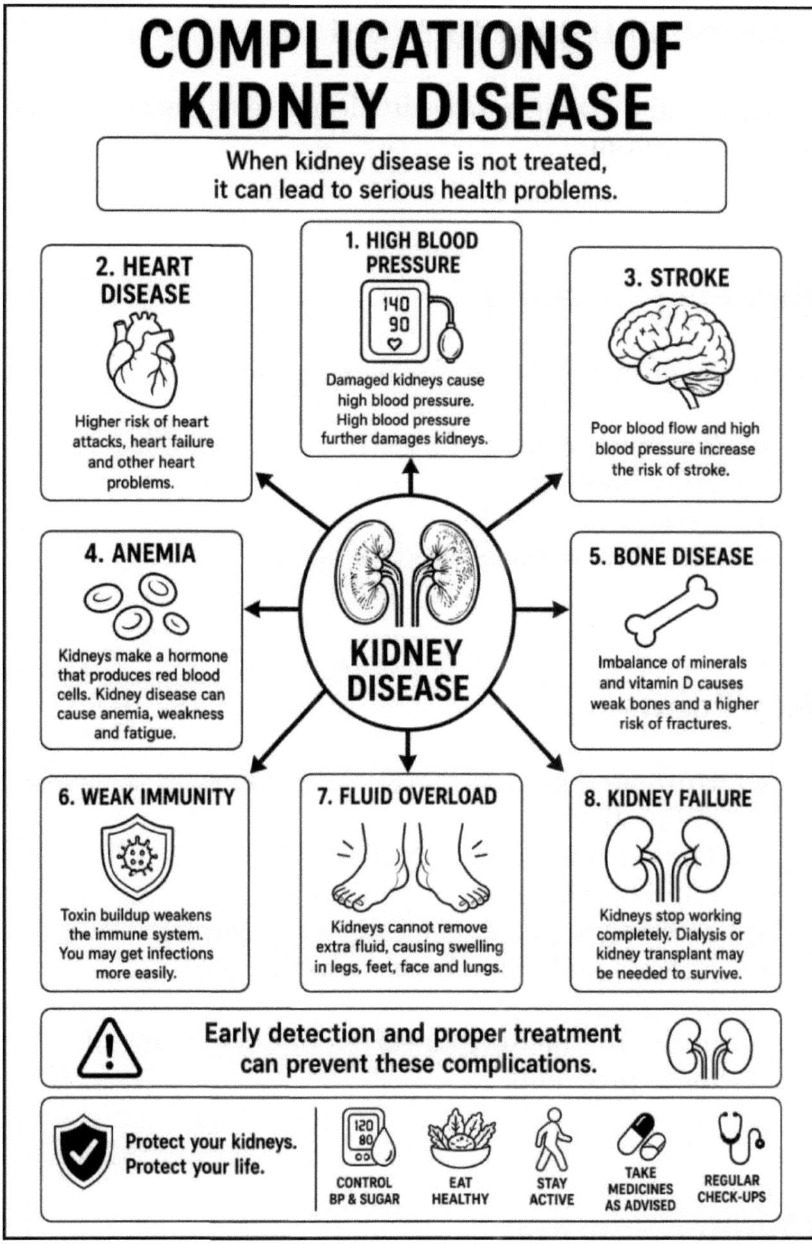
COMPLICATIONS OF KIDNEY DISEASE
When kidney disease is not treated, it can lead to serious health problems.
1. HIGH BLOOD PRESSURE
140
90
Damaged kidneys cause high blood pressure. High blood pressure further damages kidneys.
2. HEART DISEASE
Higher risk of heart attacks, heart failure and other heart problems.
3. STROKE
Poor blood flow and high blood pressure increase the risk of stroke.
KIDNEY DISEASE
4. ANEMIA
Kidneys make a hormone that produces red blood cells. Kidney disease can cause anemia, weakness and fatigue.
5. BONE DISEASE
Imbalance of minerals and vitamin D causes weak bones and a higher risk of fractures.
6. WEAK IMMUNITY
Toxin buildup weakens the immune system. You may get infections more easily.
7. FLUID OVERLOAD
Kidneys cannot remove extra fluid, causing swelling in legs, feet, face and lungs.
8. KIDNEY FAILURE
Kidneys stop working completely. Dialysis or kidney transplant may be needed to survive.
Early detection and proper treatment can prevent these complications.
Protect your kidneys. Protect your life.
120
80
CONTROL BP & SUGAR
EAT HEALTHY
STAY ACTIVE
TAKE MEDICINES AS ADVISED
REGULAR CHECK-UPS

Common Mistake to Avoid

Ignoring mild abnormalities in kidney tests because there are no symptoms.

Red Flag Warning

Seek urgent medical care if you experience:

- Severe shortness of breath
- Rapid swelling
- Persistent vomiting
- Extreme weakness or confusion

Key Points

- Untreated kidney disease leads to progressive loss of function
- The heart is commonly affected
- Fluid overload can impair breathing
- Electrolyte imbalance can be dangerous
- Anemia and bone disease are frequent complications
- Early treatment can prevent or delay many of these problems

---

Chapter Summary

When kidney disease is not properly managed, it can lead to serious complications affecting the heart, lungs, blood, bones, and overall health. These changes develop gradually but can become life-threatening over time.

The most important message is that many of these complications are preventable. Early detection, regular monitoring, and consistent treatment can significantly improve outcomes and preserve quality of life.

Action Plan

- Do not ignore abnormal kidney test results
- Maintain regular follow-up with your doctor
- Control blood pressure and blood sugar carefully
- Report new symptoms early
- Follow dietary and medication advice consistently

Transition to the Next Chapter

Now that you understand what can happen if kidney disease is not controlled, the next step is to learn how it is diagnosed and monitored. In the next chapter, we will look at the simple tests that help detect kidney problems early and guide treatment.

CHAPTER 6: How Kidney Disease Is Found and Followed

Why You Cannot Rely on Symptoms

Most kidney problems are not discovered because of symptoms. They are found because someone takes the time to look.

That may be during a routine checkup, a diabetes visit, a blood pressure follow-up, or even a pre-operative evaluation. A simple set of tests can reveal changes long before the body begins to complain.

This is an important shift in thinking.

Kidney disease is usually detected in the laboratory, not in how you feel.

If you wait for symptoms, you may miss the stage where action is most effective.

Who Should Be Tested Regularly

Not everyone needs frequent testing, but many people should not miss it.

Regular kidney testing is especially important if you have:

- Diabetes

- High blood pressure
- Heart disease
- A family history of kidney disease
- Recurrent kidney stones
- Age beyond midlife

These are common situations. That is exactly why routine testing becomes so valuable.

A simple plan, done consistently, can detect problems early and guide timely care.

Blood Tests: The First Window

The most common starting point is a blood test called **serum creatinine**.

Creatinine is a waste product from normal muscle activity. Healthy kidneys remove it from the blood.

When kidney function declines:

- Creatinine rises

But one number alone does not tell the full story. Creatinine is influenced by age, body size, and muscle mass. A muscular person may naturally have a higher value than someone smaller or older.

So we do not interpret creatinine in isolation.

---

eGFR: Turning Numbers Into Meaning

To make better sense of kidney function, we use the **estimated glomerular filtration rate**, or eGFR.

This value is calculated from creatinine along with age and other factors. It gives a clearer picture of how well the kidneys are filtering blood.

In practical terms:

- Higher eGFR suggests better kidney function
- Lower eGFR indicates reduced function

Doctors use eGFR to:

- Detect kidney disease early
- Understand how advanced it is
- Follow changes over time

More important than any single reading is the trend. A stable value over years is reassuring. A steady decline needs attention.

Urine Tests: Finding Problems Early

Urine testing is simple, inexpensive, and very informative.

It can reveal problems even when blood tests are still normal.

Key findings include:

- **Protein or albumin in urine**, an early sign of kidney damage

- **Blood in urine**, which may point to several conditions
- **Signs of infection or inflammation**

In people with diabetes or high blood pressure, a small amount of protein in the urine may be the first indication that the kidneys are under stress.

Looking at Structure: Imaging

Sometimes we need to look at the kidneys themselves, not just how they function.

Imaging tests help with this.

Common options include:

- **Ultrasound**, which is safe and widely available
- **CT scan**, which provides more detailed images when needed

These tests can show:

- Kidney size and shape
- Presence of stones
- Obstruction to urine flow
- Structural abnormalities

They are especially useful when the cause of kidney dysfunction is not clear.

HOW KIDNEY DISEASE IS DIAGNOSED

Doctors use tests to check how well your kidneys are working and find the cause of the problem.

1. BLOOD TESTS

- Check kidney function (creatinine, eGFR)
- Check electrolytes
- Check for anemia

2. URINE TESTS

- Check for protein or blood in urine
- Check for infection
- Check how concentrated your urine is

3. IMAGING TESTS

- Ultrasound of kidneys
- Check size, shape and structure
- Detect stones, blockage or other problems

4. OTHER TESTS (IF NEEDED)

- Kidney biopsy (tissue test) to find the exact cause
- Special blood tests for autoimmune diseases

5. RESULTS HELP DOCTORS

- Find the cause of kidney disease
- Check how well kidneys are working
- Determine the stage and severity
- Plan the right treatment
- Monitor progress over time

Early diagnosis helps in early treatment, slows down kidney damage and protects your health.

When a Biopsy Is Needed

In certain situations, more precise information is required.

A **kidney biopsy** involves taking a small sample of kidney tissue and examining it under a microscope.

It is usually considered when:

- The diagnosis is uncertain
- A specific disease is suspected
- Treatment decisions depend on exact findings

Although it may sound intimidating, it is a carefully performed procedure that provides valuable information when needed.

Staging Chronic Kidney Disease

Once kidney disease is identified, it is often grouped into stages based on eGFR and urine findings.

This helps guide:

- Treatment decisions
- Frequency of follow-up
- Long-term planning

In simple terms:

- Early stages may have no symptoms
- Later stages indicate more significant loss of function

The stage is not just a label. It is a guide to what should be done next.

A Practical Example

A patient with long-standing high blood pressure comes for routine testing.

Results show:

- Slightly elevated creatinine
- Mildly reduced eGFR
- Small amount of protein in urine

This is early kidney disease.

At this stage:

- Blood pressure control is improved
- Medications are adjusted
- Follow-up is planned

Because the problem is found early, there is a real opportunity to slow its progress.

Doctor's Pearl

Kidney disease is often discovered in routine tests. Do not skip them.

Common Mistake to Avoid

Waiting for symptoms before getting kidney function tested.

Red Flag Warning

Seek medical advice if tests show:

- Rising creatinine over time
- Falling eGFR
- Persistent protein or blood in urine

Key Points

- Kidney disease is usually detected through tests, not symptoms
- Creatinine is a starting point but needs context
- eGFR gives a clearer picture of kidney function
- Urine tests can detect early damage
- Imaging helps identify structural problems
- Staging guides treatment and follow-up

Chapter Summary

Kidney disease is most often found through simple blood and urine tests rather than symptoms. Creatinine and eGFR provide insight into kidney function, while urine tests can reveal early signs of damage. Imaging and, in selected cases, biopsy help identify the cause.

The most important message is that early detection is possible. With regular testing, especially in those at higher risk, kidney disease can be identified at a stage when meaningful action can be taken.

Action Plan

• Get regular blood tests, including creatinine and eGFR, if you are at risk
• Do periodic urine testing to check for protein and other changes
• Keep a record of your results and watch trends over time
• Discuss your reports with your doctor in detail
• Follow the recommended schedule for repeat testing

Transition to the Next Chapter

Now that you understand how kidney disease is detected, the next step is to learn how to read these results without fear. In the next chapter, we will make sense of kidney numbers in a simple and practical way.

CHAPTER 7: Understanding Your Kidney Numbers Without Fear

From Confusion to Clarity

I have seen this many times.

A patient receives a lab report, glances at a few numbers, and immediately becomes anxious. Words like creatinine, eGFR, and protein in urine sound technical and unfamiliar. It is easy to assume something serious is wrong.

Let me reassure you.

These numbers are not meant to frighten you. They are meant to guide you.

Once you understand what they represent, they become tools that help you take control of your health.

Creatinine: Useful, But Not the Whole Story

Creatinine is a waste product that comes from normal muscle activity. The kidneys remove it from the blood.

When kidney function declines:

- Creatinine tends to rise

This sounds straightforward, but there is an important detail.

Creatinine varies between individuals.

It depends on:

- Age
- Body size
- Muscle mass

A younger or more muscular person may naturally have a higher creatinine than an older or smaller individual.

So, one number by itself does not define your kidney health.

---

eGFR: A Better Measure of Function

To better understand kidney performance, we use **eGFR**, or estimated glomerular filtration rate.

This value is calculated using creatinine along with age and other factors. It gives a more practical sense of how well your kidneys are filtering blood.

In simple terms:

- Higher eGFR means better kidney function
- Lower eGFR means reduced function

Doctors rely on this number to assess kidney health and follow changes over time.

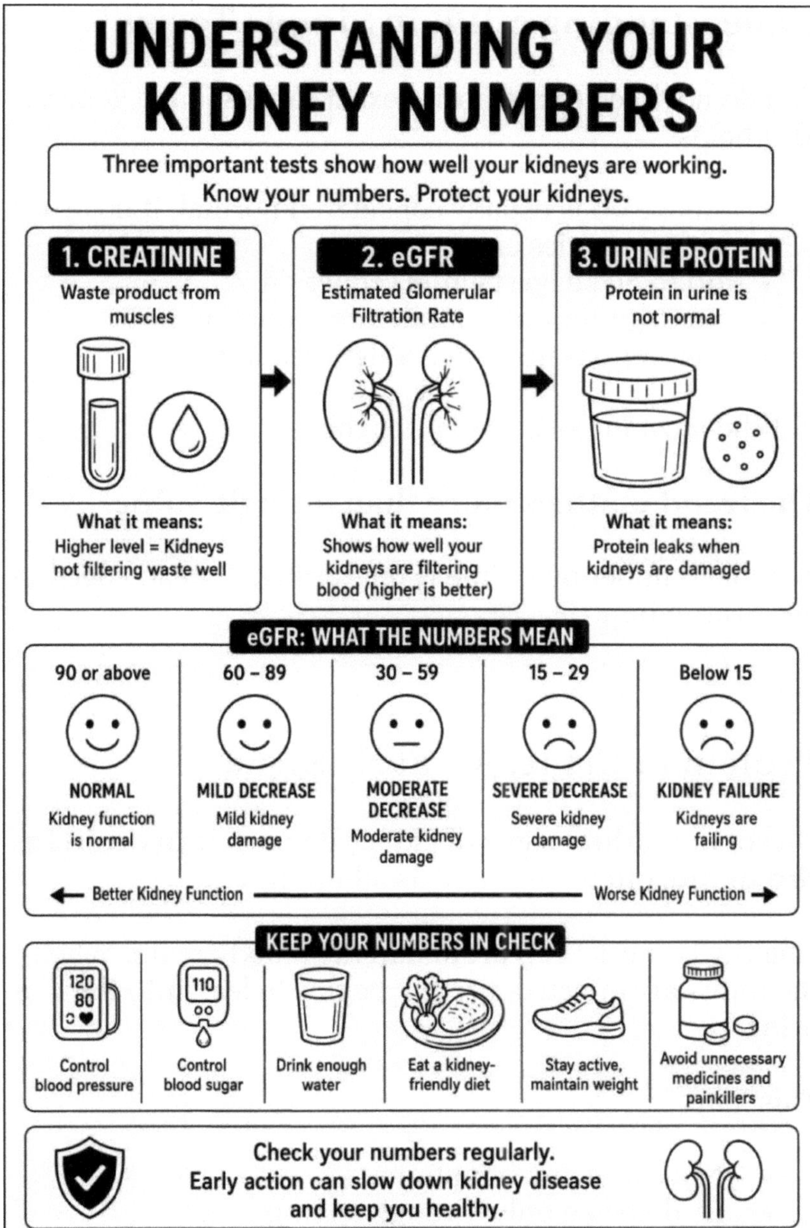
UNDERSTANDING YOUR KIDNEY NUMBERS
Three important tests show how well your kidneys are working.
Know your numbers. Protect your kidneys.
1. CREATININE
Waste product from muscles
What it means:
Higher level = Kidneys not filtering waste well
2. eGFR
Estimated Glomerular Filtration Rate
What it means:
Shows how well your kidneys are filtering blood (higher is better)
3. URINE PROTEIN
Protein in urine is not normal
What it means:
Protein leaks when kidneys are damaged
eGFR: WHAT THE NUMBERS MEAN
90 or above
NORMAL
Kidney function is normal
60 – 89
MILD DECREASE
Mild kidney damage
30 – 59
MODERATE DECREASE
Moderate kidney damage
15 – 29
SEVERE DECREASE
Severe kidney damage
Below 15
KIDNEY FAILURE
Kidneys are failing
Better Kidney Function
Worse Kidney Function
KEEP YOUR NUMBERS IN CHECK
120
80
Control blood pressure
110
Control blood sugar
Drink enough water
Eat a kidney-friendly diet
Stay active, maintain weight
Avoid unnecessary medicines and painkillers
Check your numbers regularly.
Early action can slow down kidney disease and keep you healthy.

Understanding eGFR in Simple Terms

You do not need to memorize exact ranges, but a general idea helps.

- Above 90 is usually considered normal, if no other abnormalities exist
- 60 to 89 suggests mild reduction
- 30 to 59 indicates moderate reduction
- Below 30 reflects more significant loss

But the most important point is this:

The trend matters more than a single value.

A stable number over time is reassuring. A steady decline needs attention.

Protein in Urine: An Early Signal

One of the earliest signs of kidney damage is **protein in the urine**, often measured as albumin.

Healthy kidneys keep protein in the bloodstream. When the filters are affected, protein begins to leak into the urine.

This may:

- Not cause any symptoms
- Be detected only through testing

Even small amounts can be important, especially in people with diabetes or high blood pressure.

Other Numbers You May See

Kidney disease can affect several other laboratory values.

You may notice changes in:

- **Potassium**, which influences heart rhythm
- **Sodium**, which affects fluid balance
- **Bicarbonate**, related to acid balance
- **Hemoglobin**, which may fall due to anemia

These values help your doctor understand how kidney disease is affecting your body as a whole.

Why Trends Tell the Real Story

Let me emphasize something that can save you a great deal of unnecessary worry.

A single abnormal report does not define your condition.

Doctors look for:

- Patterns over time
- Consistency across tests
- The overall clinical picture

For example:

- A slightly elevated creatinine that remains stable may not be serious
- A gradual rise over time deserves attention

- A sudden change may indicate an acute problem

Understanding this prevents overreaction.

Common Misunderstandings

There are a few misconceptions that create unnecessary anxiety.

- A mildly abnormal creatinine does not mean dialysis is near
- A normal creatinine does not always rule out early kidney disease
- eGFR may decline slightly with age
- Numbers must always be interpreted in context

Clearing these misunderstandings makes a big difference.

A Practical Example

A patient comes in worried about a slightly high creatinine.

He assumes the worst.

On reviewing past records, we find:

- The value has been stable for several years
- eGFR has not changed significantly
- Urine tests are normal

This is not a rapidly progressing condition. It is a stable situation that requires monitoring, not panic.

This is why interpretation matters.

Doctor's Pearl

Do not react to a single number. Look at the pattern over time.

Common Mistake to Avoid

Comparing your lab results with someone else's instead of your own previous reports.

Red Flag Warning

Seek medical advice if you notice:

- Rising creatinine over time
- Declining eGFR
- Increasing protein in urine
- Abnormal potassium levels

Key Points

- Lab values are tools for guidance, not sources of fear

- Creatinine must be interpreted in context
- eGFR gives a clearer picture of kidney function
- Protein in urine is an early warning sign
- Trends over time are more important than single values
- Proper interpretation prevents unnecessary anxiety

Chapter Summary

Understanding kidney-related lab values helps you take an active role in your care. Creatinine and eGFR provide insight into kidney function, while urine protein can reveal early damage. Other values reflect how kidney disease affects the body.

The key principle is to focus on trends rather than isolated numbers. With regular monitoring and proper interpretation, these tests become powerful tools that guide treatment and protect long-term health.

Action Plan

• Keep a record of your kidney test results
• Focus on trends over time rather than single values
• Discuss your reports with your doctor
• Avoid unnecessary worry over minor variations
• Follow medical advice based on the overall picture

Transition to the Next Chapter

Now that you understand your kidney numbers, the next step is to look at the most common form of kidney disease. In the next chapter, we will discuss chronic kidney disease, how it develops, and how it can be managed over time.

CHAPTER 8: Chronic Kidney Disease: The Condition That Often Stays Hidden

A Slow and Quiet Process

Chronic kidney disease, often called CKD, is not something that appears suddenly.

It develops gradually, usually over many years. In the early stages, it does not cause noticeable symptoms. That is why many people live with it without knowing.

CKD is generally defined as:

- Reduced kidney function, or
- Evidence of kidney damage, such as protein in the urine
- Present for at least three months

The key idea is persistence.

A temporary change in kidney function is not the same as chronic disease. CKD reflects an ongoing process that deserves attention.

Why So Many People Are Unaware

CKD is common, but awareness is low.

There are simple reasons for this:

- It progresses slowly
- Early stages are silent
- Testing is not always done regularly
- Mild abnormalities are often overlooked

As a result, many people continue their normal lives while kidney function declines quietly.

This is not due to neglect. It is simply the nature of the disease.

The Most Common Causes

In everyday practice, most cases of CKD are linked to a few conditions.

Diabetes
Long-term high blood sugar damages the tiny filtering units of the kidneys.

High Blood Pressure
Constant pressure affects the blood vessels inside the kidneys.

Other contributing factors include:

- Long-term use of certain medications
- Repeated infections
- Obstruction from stones or prostate problems
- Autoimmune conditions
- Genetic disorders such as polycystic kidney disease

Often, more than one factor is involved.

STAGES OF CHRONIC KIDNEY DISEASE (CKD)

CKD has 5 stages. The lower the eGFR, the more severe the kidney damage.

STAGE	eGFR	WHAT IT MEANS	WHAT TO EXPECT
STAGE 1 NORMAL OR HIGH	90 or above	**Normal kidney function** Kidneys are working well.	Keep kidneys healthy with a healthy lifestyle.
STAGE 2 MILD DECREASE	60 – 89	**Mild kidney damage** Kidneys are still working well, but there is some damage.	Treat underlying conditions. Regular check-ups are important.
STAGE 3 MODERATE DECREASE	30 – 59	**Moderate kidney damage** Kidneys are not working as well as before.	Follow treatment, diet and medicine. Slow down kidney damage.
STAGE 4 SEVERE DECREASE	15 – 29	**Severe kidney damage** Kidneys are working very little.	Prepare for kidney replacement treatment. Close monitoring needed.
STAGE 5 KIDNEY FAILURE	Below 15	**Kidney failure** Kidneys can no longer work.	Dialysis or kidney transplant is needed to survive.

EARLY DETECTION AND PROPER CARE CAN SLOW DOWN CKD PROGRESSION.

How CKD Progresses

A common question is, "Will it keep getting worse?"

The answer is not the same for everyone.

In some people:

- Kidney function declines very slowly
- It may remain stable for years

In others:

- Decline may be faster

What makes the difference?

- Control of blood sugar
- Control of blood pressure
- Amount of protein in urine
- Lifestyle habits such as diet, weight, and smoking

The encouraging part is that many of these factors can be improved.

Early Stage Versus Advanced Stage

In early CKD:

- You feel normal
- Abnormalities appear only in tests
- There is a strong opportunity to act

In advanced CKD:

- Symptoms become noticeable
- Complications develop
- Treatment becomes more complex

This contrast highlights an important truth.

The earlier you act, the more options you have.

What Early Action Can Achieve

CKD may not always be reversible, but it is often manageable.

With proper care, you can:

- Slow progression
- Reduce complications
- Maintain a good quality of life

This usually involves:

- Controlling blood pressure
- Managing blood sugar
- Using appropriate medications
- Making lifestyle adjustments
- Monitoring regularly

These steps are simple in principle, but powerful in practice.

A Practical Clinical Situation

A patient with diabetes comes for routine evaluation.

He feels well.

Tests show:

- Mild reduction in kidney function
- Small amount of protein in urine

At this stage:

- Blood sugar control is improved
- Blood pressure is optimized
- Follow-up is planned

Over time, kidney function remains stable.

This is a common and encouraging outcome when the problem is identified early.

Doctor’s Pearl

Chronic kidney disease is often silent, but early care can change its course.

Common Mistake to Avoid

Ignoring mild abnormalities because there are no symptoms.

Red Flag Warning

Seek medical advice if:

- Kidney function declines steadily
- Protein in urine increases
- Blood pressure becomes difficult to control

Key Points

- CKD is a slow and progressive loss of kidney function
- Early stages usually have no symptoms
- Diabetes and high blood pressure are the main causes
- Staging helps guide care
- Progression varies between individuals
- Early intervention can slow the disease

Chapter Summary

Chronic kidney disease is a common condition that develops gradually and often goes unnoticed in its early stages. Because symptoms are absent at first, it is frequently detected through routine testing. The most common causes are diabetes and high blood pressure, although other factors may contribute.

The most important message is that CKD can often be slowed. With early detection, proper treatment, and consistent lifestyle changes, many patients maintain stable kidney function and a good quality of life for years.

Action Plan

- If you have diabetes or high blood pressure, schedule regular kidney testing
- Monitor your eGFR and urine protein levels
- Follow medical advice consistently
- Maintain a healthy lifestyle
- Do not ignore early abnormalities

Transition to the Next Chapter

While chronic kidney disease develops slowly, some kidney problems occur suddenly and require urgent attention. In the next chapter, we will discuss acute kidney injury and how it can often be reversed with timely treatment.

CHAPTER 9: Acute Kidney Injury: When Things Change Quickly

A Sudden Shift in Kidney Function

So far, we have focused on kidney problems that develop slowly over time.

Acute kidney injury, or AKI, is very different.

Here, the change is sudden.

A person who was doing reasonably well may, within a short period of time, develop abnormal kidney function. This can happen over hours or a few days. The body does not have time to adjust, and that is what makes this condition important.

The encouraging part is this:

In many cases, acute kidney injury can be reversed if treated early.

What Happens Inside the Body

In AKI, the kidneys suddenly lose their ability to do their usual work.

As a result:

- Waste products begin to accumulate
- Fluid balance becomes disturbed
- Electrolytes may become unstable

Because this change is rapid, the effects can be felt more quickly than in chronic kidney disease.

The problem is not only the loss of function, but the speed at which it occurs.

The Three Common Causes

Most cases of acute kidney injury fall into three broad categories.

Reduced Blood Flow to the Kidneys

The kidneys depend on a steady supply of blood.

When this drops, function declines.

This can happen with:

- Dehydration from vomiting or diarrhea
- Severe blood loss
- Low blood pressure
- Heart problems

Direct Injury to Kidney Tissue

Sometimes the kidneys themselves are affected.

This may occur due to:

- Severe infections
- Certain medications
- Contrast agents used in imaging
- Inflammatory conditions

Obstruction to Urine Flow

If urine cannot flow out normally, pressure builds up and damages the kidneys.

Common causes include:

- Kidney stones
- Enlarged prostate
- Blockage in the urinary tract

Relieving the obstruction often improves kidney function.

Situations Where AKI Is Common

Acute kidney injury often occurs in certain situations.

These include:

- Severe dehydration
- Serious infections
- Hospitalization for major illness
- Surgery
- Use of certain medications

Being aware of these situations can help in prevention.

Symptoms: Not Always Obvious

AKI does not always produce clear symptoms.

In some cases:

- There may be very little to notice

In others, you may experience:

- Reduced urine output
- Swelling
- Fatigue
- Nausea or vomiting
- Confusion in severe cases

Because symptoms can be mild or unclear, blood tests are often needed to confirm the diagnosis.

How It Is Diagnosed

Doctors recognize AKI by:

- A rise in creatinine over a short period
- A decrease in urine output

But identifying AKI is only the first step.

The next step is to find the cause.

This may involve:

- Reviewing medications
- Checking hydration status
- Performing blood and urine tests
- Using imaging when needed

The goal is to correct the underlying problem quickly.

Treatment: Focus on the Cause

Treatment of AKI depends on what caused it.

Common approaches include:

- Giving fluids if dehydration is present
- Treating infections promptly
- Stopping or adjusting harmful medications
- Relieving obstruction

In many cases, kidney function improves once the cause is addressed.

In more severe cases:

- Temporary dialysis may be needed

Prevention: Often Within Your Control

Many cases of AKI can be prevented.

Simple steps include:

- Staying well hydrated, especially during illness
- Avoiding unnecessary use of certain medications
- Informing your doctor about kidney issues before procedures
- Monitoring kidney function during high-risk situations

These measures are particularly important for older individuals and those with existing kidney disease.

A Practical Example

An elderly patient develops diarrhea during hot weather and becomes dehydrated.

He continues his regular medications, including blood pressure drugs and occasional pain medicine.

Within a few days:

- He feels weak
- Urine output decreases
- Blood tests show worsening kidney function

With proper treatment, including fluids and medication adjustment, kidney function improves.

This is a common and often preventable situation.

Doctor's Pearl

Acute kidney injury is often reversible if recognized and treated early.

Common Mistake to Avoid

Continuing medications during dehydration or illness without guidance.

Red Flag Warning

Seek urgent care if you notice:

- Sudden decrease in urine
- Severe weakness or confusion
- Persistent vomiting
- Rapid swelling

Key Points

- AKI is a sudden decline in kidney function
- It develops over hours to days
- Common causes include dehydration, infection, medications, and obstruction
- Symptoms may be mild or severe
- Early treatment can lead to recovery
- Prevention is often possible

Chapter Summary

Acute kidney injury is a sudden and potentially serious decline in kidney function. Unlike chronic kidney disease, it develops quickly and, in many cases, can be reversed with timely treatment. The most common causes include reduced blood flow, direct injury to the kidneys, and obstruction to urine flow.

The key to managing AKI is early recognition and prompt treatment. Awareness of risk factors and preventive measures can significantly reduce its occurrence.

Action Plan

• Stay well hydrated, especially during illness
• Avoid unnecessary or excessive use of medications that may harm the kidneys
• Inform your doctor about all medicines you are taking
• Seek medical attention early if symptoms develop
• Monitor kidney function if you are at higher risk

Transition to the Next Chapter

Now that you understand both chronic and acute kidney conditions, the next step is to focus on the two most important causes of kidney damage. In the next chapter, we will discuss how diabetes and high blood pressure affect the kidneys and how controlling them can protect your health.

CHAPTER 10: Diabetes and High Blood Pressure: The Two Biggest Threats to Your Kidneys

Why These Two Conditions Matter So Much

If there is one message I want every reader to remember, it is this:

Most kidney disease is not random. It has clear, common causes.

In everyday medical practice, two conditions account for the majority of cases:

- Diabetes
- High blood pressure

They are extremely common. They often remain silent for years. And when not well controlled, they slowly damage the kidneys.

The important part is this:

Both conditions are manageable.
When controlled well, they protect the kidneys.
When ignored, they quietly damage them.

How Diabetes Damages the Kidneys

In diabetes, blood sugar levels remain higher than normal over long periods.

This affects the kidneys in a gradual but steady way.

Inside the kidneys are tiny filtering units. These filters are delicate and highly sensitive to changes in blood chemistry.

Over time:

- High sugar levels damage these filters
- The filtering walls become less effective
- Protein begins to leak into the urine
- Kidney function slowly declines

This process is called diabetic kidney disease.

The Early Stage: No Symptoms

In the beginning:

- There are no symptoms
- The person feels normal
- Only tests reveal the problem

A small amount of protein in the urine may be the first sign.

At this stage, there is a major opportunity.

With proper care:

- Blood sugar can be improved

- Blood pressure can be controlled
- Medications can protect the kidneys

Early action can slow or even stabilize the condition.

How High Blood Pressure Affects the Kidneys

High blood pressure places constant stress on blood vessels.

In the kidneys:

- It damages the small arteries
- Reduces effective blood flow
- Leads to gradual loss of function

This damage builds slowly over time.

There is also a cycle:

- Kidney disease makes blood pressure harder to control
- Uncontrolled blood pressure further damages the kidneys

Breaking this cycle is essential.

The Two Conditions Often Work Together

In many patients, diabetes and high blood pressure are present together.

When this happens:

- The risk to the kidneys increases significantly
- Damage may progress faster

This is why both conditions must be managed together, not separately.

Who Is at Higher Risk

Not everyone with diabetes or high blood pressure will develop kidney disease, but certain factors increase the risk.

These include:

- Long duration of disease
- Poor control of blood sugar or blood pressure
- Presence of protein in urine
- Smoking
- Excess body weight

The longer these factors continue, the greater the risk.

What You Can Do to Protect Your Kidneys

The most encouraging part of this chapter is that much of the risk can be reduced.

Control Blood Sugar

- Follow dietary advice

- Take medications as prescribed
- Monitor regularly

Control Blood Pressure

- Keep readings within target range
- Monitor at home if possible

Use Protective Medications

- Certain medicines help reduce stress on the kidneys
- They also reduce protein loss in urine

Adopt Healthy Habits

- Reduce salt intake
- Maintain a healthy weight
- Stay physically active

These steps are simple but powerful.

A Practical Clinical Example

A patient with diabetes comes for routine follow-up.

He feels well.

Tests show:

- Mild protein in urine
- Slight reduction in kidney function

At this stage:

- Blood sugar control is improved
- Blood pressure is adjusted
- Medications are optimized

Over time, kidney function remains stable.

This is the outcome we aim for.

Doctor's Pearl

The best protection for your kidneys is consistent control of diabetes and blood pressure.

Common Mistake to Avoid

Thinking that "slightly high" blood sugar or blood pressure is not important.

Red Flag Warning

Seek medical attention if:

- Blood pressure remains high despite treatment
- Protein in urine increases
- Kidney function declines on repeated tests

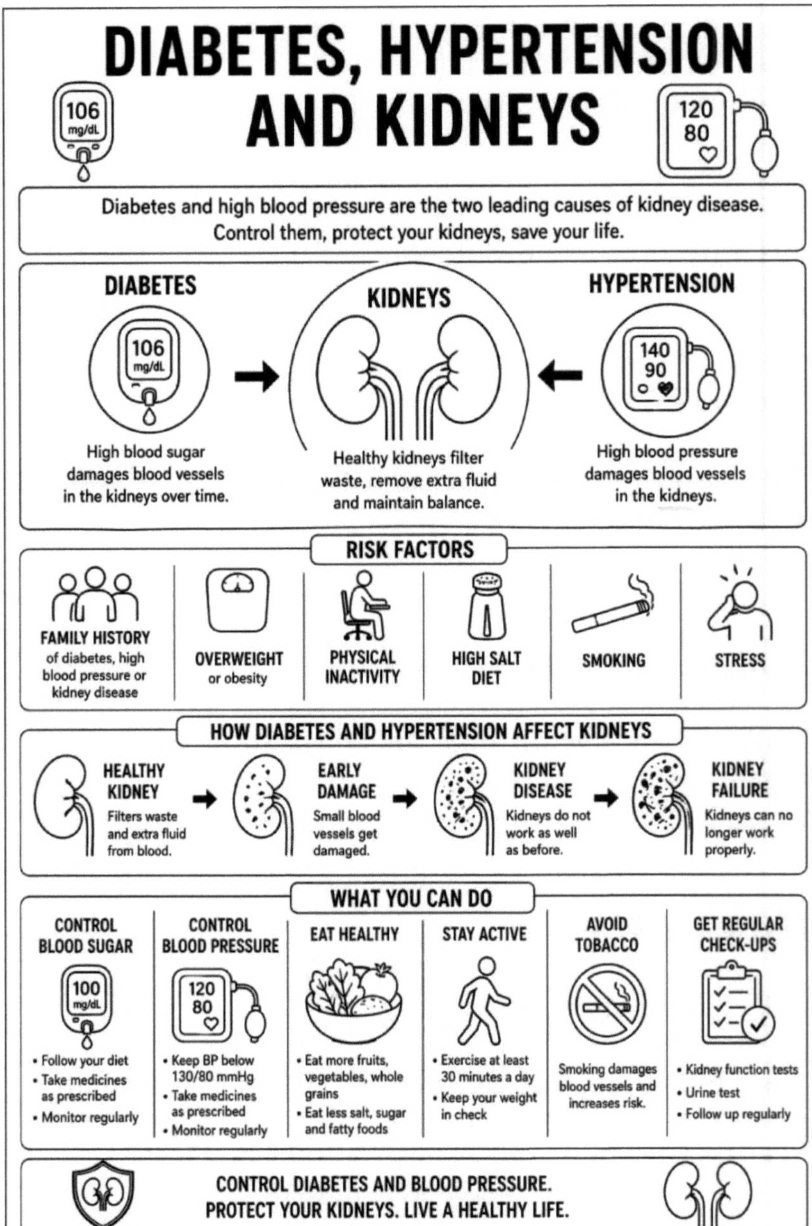

DIABETES, HYPERTENSION AND KIDNEYS
106 mg/dL
120 80
Diabetes and high blood pressure are the two leading causes of kidney disease.
Control them, protect your kidneys, save your life.
DIABETES
106 mg/dL
High blood sugar damages blood vessels in the kidneys over time.
KIDNEYS
Healthy kidneys filter waste, remove extra fluid and maintain balance.
HYPERTENSION
140 90
High blood pressure damages blood vessels in the kidneys.
RISK FACTORS
FAMILY HISTORY of diabetes, high blood pressure or kidney disease
OVERWEIGHT or obesity
PHYSICAL INACTIVITY
HIGH SALT DIET
SMOKING
STRESS
HOW DIABETES AND HYPERTENSION AFFECT KIDNEYS
HEALTHY KIDNEY
Filters waste and extra fluid from blood.
EARLY DAMAGE
Small blood vessels get damaged.
KIDNEY DISEASE
Kidneys do not work as well as before.
KIDNEY FAILURE
Kidneys can no longer work properly.
WHAT YOU CAN DO
CONTROL BLOOD SUGAR
100 mg/dL
• Follow your diet
• Take medicines as prescribed
• Monitor regularly
CONTROL BLOOD PRESSURE
120 80
• Keep BP below 130/80 mmHg
• Take medicines as prescribed
• Monitor regularly
EAT HEALTHY
• Eat more fruits, vegetables, whole grains
• Eat less salt, sugar and fatty foods
STAY ACTIVE
• Exercise at least 30 minutes a day
• Keep your weight in check
AVOID TOBACCO
Smoking damages blood vessels and increases risk.
GET REGULAR CHECK-UPS
• Kidney function tests
• Urine test
• Follow up regularly
CONTROL DIABETES AND BLOOD PRESSURE.
PROTECT YOUR KIDNEYS. LIVE A HEALTHY LIFE.

Key Points

- Diabetes and high blood pressure are the leading causes of kidney disease
- Damage develops slowly and often without symptoms
- Protein in urine is an early warning sign
- Good control can slow progression
- Lifestyle and medication both play a role

Chapter Summary

Diabetes and high blood pressure are the most common causes of kidney disease. Both conditions gradually damage the blood vessels and filters within the kidneys, leading to progressive loss of function.

The key message is that this damage is not inevitable. With early detection, proper treatment, and consistent lifestyle changes, many patients can slow progression and maintain kidney health for years.

Action Plan

- Monitor blood sugar regularly if you have diabetes
- Keep blood pressure within target range
- Take medications as prescribed
- Get regular kidney tests
- Maintain a healthy lifestyle

Transition to the Next Chapter

While diabetes and high blood pressure are the most common causes, they are not the only ones. In the next chapter, we will explore other kidney diseases that you should be aware of and how they present.

CHAPTER 11: Other Kidney Diseases You Should Not Overlook

Looking Beyond the Usual Causes

By now, you understand that diabetes and high blood pressure are the leading causes of kidney disease.

But medicine is never limited to just two explanations.

There are several other kidney conditions that, although less common, are very important. Some affect younger individuals. Some present with unusual symptoms. Some require completely different treatment approaches.

If we focus only on the common causes, we may miss these conditions.

That is why it is important to keep a broader perspective.

Glomerulonephritis: When the Filters Are Inflamed

Inside the kidneys are millions of tiny filters called glomeruli.

In **glomerulonephritis**, these filters become inflamed.

This inflammation may occur due to:

- Immune system disorders
- Infections
- Systemic diseases affecting the whole body

Patients may notice:

- Blood in urine
- Protein in urine
- Swelling
- Sometimes high blood pressure

In some cases, the condition can progress quickly.

Early diagnosis is essential because treatment often depends on identifying the exact cause.

Kidney Infections: More Than a Simple Urinary Infection

Many people are familiar with bladder infections.

But when an infection reaches the kidneys, it becomes more serious. This is called **kidney infection** or pyelonephritis.

Common features include:

- Fever and chills
- Pain in the back or side
- Burning during urination
- Nausea or vomiting

With prompt treatment, most patients recover well.

However, repeated infections or delayed treatment can lead to long-term damage.

Polycystic Kidney Disease: A Genetic Condition

Polycystic kidney disease is a condition that often runs in families.

In this disorder:

- Multiple fluid-filled cysts develop in the kidneys
- The kidneys gradually enlarge
- Normal kidney tissue is replaced over time

Patients may develop:

- High blood pressure
- Abdominal discomfort
- Declining kidney function

Family history plays an important role. Early screening in at-risk individuals can help detect the condition sooner.

Obstruction: When Urine Flow Is Blocked

The kidneys depend on a free flow of urine.

When this flow is blocked:

- Pressure builds up inside the kidneys
- Kidney function is affected

Common causes include:

- Kidney stones
- Enlarged prostate
- Narrowing of urinary passages

One important point to remember:

Obstruction is often reversible if treated early.

Delay can lead to permanent damage.

Drug-Related Kidney Injury: A Preventable Cause

Certain medications can affect kidney function, especially when:

- Used frequently
- Taken in high doses
- Used without proper monitoring

Common examples include:

- Pain medications such as NSAIDs
- Some antibiotics
- Contrast agents used in imaging

This is one of the most preventable causes of kidney damage.

Awareness and careful use of medicines can avoid many problems.

Autoimmune and Systemic Diseases

Some conditions affect multiple organs, including the kidneys.

These include:

- Lupus
- Vasculitis
- Other immune-related disorders

In these diseases:

- The immune system mistakenly attacks kidney tissue
- Damage can occur if not treated early

Management often requires specialist care.

Less Common but Important Conditions

There are other kidney-related conditions that are less frequently seen but still important.

These include:

- Congenital abnormalities present from birth
- Rare metabolic disorders
- Kidney tumors

While uncommon, they should be considered when symptoms or test results do not fit usual patterns.

A Real-Life Example

A young patient presents with swelling and blood in urine.

He has no diabetes. No high blood pressure.

Further evaluation reveals glomerulonephritis.

With early treatment, kidney function improves.

This case highlights an important point.

Not all kidney disease follows the same pattern.

Doctor's Pearl

When symptoms are unusual, look beyond the common causes.

Common Mistake to Avoid

Ignoring blood in urine because there is no pain.

Red Flag Warning

Seek medical attention if you notice:

- Blood in urine
- Persistent fever with urinary symptoms
- Severe flank pain
- Unexplained swelling

Key Points

- Several kidney diseases exist beyond diabetes and hypertension
- Glomerulonephritis involves inflammation of kidney filters
- Kidney infections can cause serious damage if untreated
- Obstruction can impair kidney function but is often reversible
- Some medications can harm the kidneys
- Early diagnosis improves outcomes

Chapter Summary

Kidney disease is not limited to common causes such as diabetes and high blood pressure. A range of other conditions, including inflammatory diseases, infections, genetic disorders, obstruction, and medication-related injury, can affect the kidneys.

Recognizing these conditions early is essential, especially when symptoms do not follow typical patterns. With timely diagnosis and appropriate treatment, many of these diseases can be effectively managed.

Action Plan

- Do not ignore unusual symptoms such as blood in urine
- Seek evaluation for persistent urinary or systemic symptoms
- Use medications carefully and under medical guidance
- Inform your doctor about any family history of kidney disease
- Follow up regularly if any abnormality is detected

Transition to the Next Chapter

Now that you understand the different types of kidney diseases, the next step is to focus on what you can do every day to protect your kidneys. In the next chapter, we will look at simple lifestyle habits that make a lasting difference.

CHAPTER 12: Daily Habits That Protect Your Kidneys for Life

Where Real Protection Begins

After discussing diseases, tests, and treatments, we now come to something far more powerful.

Your daily habits.

Medicines help. Procedures help. But what truly shapes long-term kidney health is what you do every single day.

What you eat.
How active you are.
How well you control your health conditions.
How consistently you follow through.

These may sound simple, but they are not small. They are the foundation of everything we have discussed so far.

Keep It Practical, Not Perfect

Many people feel overwhelmed when they hear the words "lifestyle changes."

They imagine strict diets, complicated rules, and a complete overhaul of their routine.

That approach rarely works.

What works is:

- Simple choices
- Made consistently
- That fit your daily life

You do not need perfection.

You need sustainability.

Food: Simple, Fresh, and Balanced

A kidney-friendly diet does not need to be complicated.

A practical approach includes:

- Fresh, home-cooked meals
- Plenty of vegetables
- Fruits in reasonable portions
- Whole grains in moderation
- Balanced protein intake

The focus should be on simplicity and consistency.

Avoid extremes. Avoid confusion. Stay balanced.

Salt: The One Change That Matters Most

If there is one dietary habit that makes a major difference, it is reducing salt.

Excess salt:

- Raises blood pressure
- Causes fluid retention
- Increases strain on the kidneys

Most of the salt we consume is hidden in:

- Packaged foods
- Restaurant meals
- Processed snacks

Simple steps can help:

- Cook more meals at home
- Avoid adding extra salt at the table
- Be mindful of processed foods

Even small reductions can have a meaningful long-term impact.

Protein: Balance Is the Key

Protein is essential for the body.

But very high protein intake over time can increase the workload on the kidneys.

You do not need to avoid protein.

Instead:

- Choose moderate portions
- Avoid extreme high-protein diets unless medically advised

A balanced approach supports overall health.

Hydration: Enough, Not Excess

"How much water should I drink?" is a common question.

The answer is simple, but not the same for everyone.

In general:

- Stay well hydrated
- Keep urine light in color

But remember:

- Drinking excessive amounts does not provide extra benefit
- In advanced kidney disease, fluid intake may need to be limited

So the approach should be practical and individualized.

Physical Activity: A Strong Support

Regular movement is one of the simplest and most effective ways to protect your kidneys indirectly.

It helps:

- Control blood pressure
- Improve blood sugar

- Maintain a healthy weight
- Improve overall energy

You do not need intense exercise.

Even:

- Walking
- Light daily activity
- Staying active throughout the day

can make a meaningful difference.

Consistency is more important than intensity.

Weight, Smoking, and Alcohol

These factors often work quietly in the background but have a strong effect.

Excess weight

- Increases the risk of diabetes and high blood pressure

Smoking

- Damages blood vessels and accelerates kidney damage

Alcohol

- Can affect blood pressure and hydration if taken in excess

A balanced and moderate approach is always better than extremes.

Sleep and Stress: Often Overlooked

Sleep and stress also influence health.

Poor sleep and chronic stress can:

- Affect blood pressure
- Influence blood sugar
- Reduce overall well-being

Simple habits help:

- Maintain a regular sleep schedule
- Allow time for rest and relaxation
- Stay mentally and socially engaged

Health is not only physical. It is also mental and emotional.

A Simple Daily Routine

Let me put this into a practical example.

Morning:

- Light, balanced breakfast
- Short walk or activity

Afternoon:

- Balanced meal
- Adequate hydration

Evening:

- Light dinner
- Avoid heavy, salty foods
- Time to unwind

There is nothing complicated here.

The strength lies in repeating it every day.

Doctor's Pearl

Small daily habits protect your kidneys more effectively than occasional big efforts.

Common Mistake to Avoid

Following extreme diets that are difficult to maintain.

Red Flag Warning

Consult your doctor before making major changes if:

- You have advanced kidney disease
- You are on fluid or dietary restrictions
- You have abnormal electrolyte levels

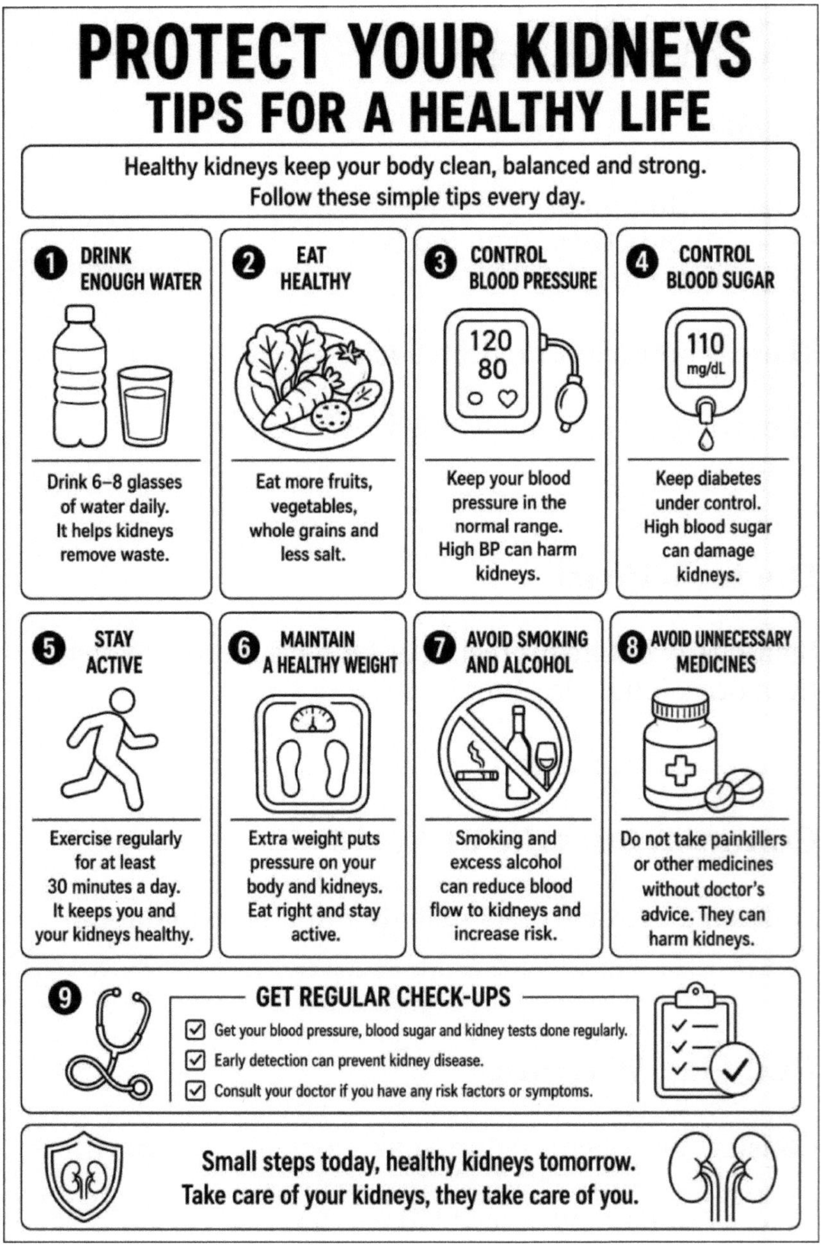

PROTECT YOUR KIDNEYS
TIPS FOR A HEALTHY LIFE
Healthy kidneys keep your body clean, balanced and strong.
Follow these simple tips every day.
1 DRINK ENOUGH WATER
Drink 6–8 glasses of water daily. It helps kidneys remove waste.
2 EAT HEALTHY
Eat more fruits, vegetables, whole grains and less salt.
3 CONTROL BLOOD PRESSURE
120
80
Keep your blood pressure in the normal range. High BP can harm kidneys.
4 CONTROL BLOOD SUGAR
110
mg/dL
Keep diabetes under control. High blood sugar can damage kidneys.
5 STAY ACTIVE
Exercise regularly for at least 30 minutes a day. It keeps you and your kidneys healthy.
6 MAINTAIN A HEALTHY WEIGHT
Extra weight puts pressure on your body and kidneys. Eat right and stay active.
7 AVOID SMOKING AND ALCOHOL
Smoking and excess alcohol can reduce blood flow to kidneys and increase risk.
8 AVOID UNNECESSARY MEDICINES
Do not take painkillers or other medicines without doctor's advice. They can harm kidneys.
9 GET REGULAR CHECK-UPS
Get your blood pressure, blood sugar and kidney tests done regularly.
Early detection can prevent kidney disease.
Consult your doctor if you have any risk factors or symptoms.
Small steps today, healthy kidneys tomorrow.
Take care of your kidneys, they take care of you.

Key Points

- Daily habits form the foundation of kidney health
- A balanced diet is more effective than strict diets
- Reducing salt is essential
- Protein intake should be moderate
- Hydration should be appropriate
- Regular activity supports overall health

Chapter Summary

Lifestyle choices play a central role in protecting kidney health. A simple and balanced approach to diet, hydration, and physical activity can significantly reduce the risk of kidney disease and slow its progression.

The goal is not perfection, but consistency. Small, steady improvements made over time have a powerful impact on long-term health.

Action Plan

• Reduce salt in your daily diet
• Eat fresh, balanced meals
• Stay adequately hydrated
• Walk or stay active regularly
• Maintain a healthy weight
• Avoid smoking and limit alcohol

Transition to the Next Chapter

While lifestyle habits form the foundation, medications also play an important role. In the next chapter, we will discuss which medicines protect your kidneys and which ones should be used with caution.

CHAPTER 13: Medicines That Help and Medicines That Harm Your Kidneys

Medicines Are Powerful, but They Must Be Used Wisely

In medical practice, medicines are among our most effective tools.

They relieve symptoms, control disease, and in many cases protect vital organs. But like all powerful tools, they must be used with care.

When used correctly, medicines can slow kidney damage and improve long-term outcomes. When used without proper guidance, they can do the opposite.

Understanding this balance is essential.

Medicines That Protect the Kidneys

Let us begin with the positive side.

There are medications that not only treat disease but also **protect kidney function**.

Blood Pressure Medicines With Added Benefit

Two groups of medicines are especially important:

- ACE inhibitors
- ARBs

These are commonly used to treat high blood pressure, but their benefit goes beyond that.

They:

- Reduce pressure within the kidney filters
- Decrease protein leakage into the urine
- Slow the progression of chronic kidney disease

For many patients, these medicines form the backbone of kidney protection.

Diabetes Medicines With Kidney Benefits

In recent years, some diabetes medications have shown clear protective effects on the kidneys.

They help by:

- Improving blood sugar control
- Reducing stress on kidney filters
- Slowing the decline in kidney function

Modern treatment now often focuses not only on controlling blood sugar but also on protecting the kidneys and heart.

This has significantly improved long-term outcomes.

Medicines That Support the Body

In addition to these, other medications help manage the effects of kidney disease.

These include:

- Diuretics to remove excess fluid
- Medicines to correct acid imbalance
- Treatments to control potassium levels
- Therapy for anemia

These medicines do not cure kidney disease, but they help maintain stability and improve quality of life.

Medicines That Can Harm the Kidneys

Now let us look at the other side.

Some medicines can affect kidney function, especially when:

- Used frequently
- Taken in high doses
- Used without monitoring

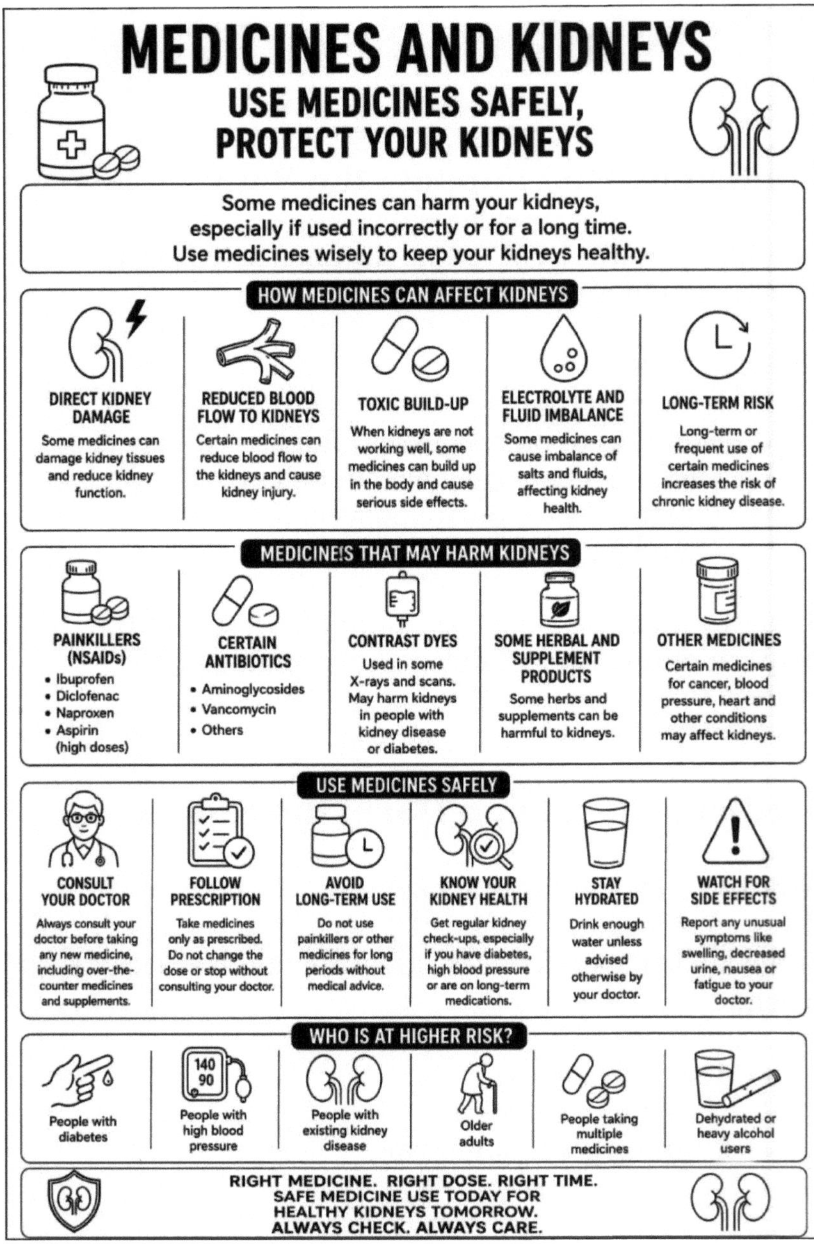
MEDICINES AND KIDNEYS
USE MEDICINES SAFELY, PROTECT YOUR KIDNEYS
Some medicines can harm your kidneys, especially if used incorrectly or for a long time. Use medicines wisely to keep your kidneys healthy.
HOW MEDICINES CAN AFFECT KIDNEYS
DIRECT KIDNEY DAMAGE
Some medicines can damage kidney tissues and reduce kidney function.
REDUCED BLOOD FLOW TO KIDNEYS
Certain medicines can reduce blood flow to the kidneys and cause kidney injury.
TOXIC BUILD-UP
When kidneys are not working well, some medicines can build up in the body and cause serious side effects.
ELECTROLYTE AND FLUID IMBALANCE
Some medicines can cause imbalance of salts and fluids, affecting kidney health.
LONG-TERM RISK
Long-term or frequent use of certain medicines increases the risk of chronic kidney disease.
MEDICINE!S THAT MAY HARM KIDNEYS
PAINKILLERS (NSAIDs)
• Ibuprofen
• Diclofenac
• Naproxen
• Aspirin (high doses)
CERTAIN ANTIBIOTICS
• Aminoglycosides
• Vancomycin
• Others
CONTRAST DYES
Used in some X-rays and scans. May harm kidneys in people with kidney disease or diabetes.
SOME HERBAL AND SUPPLEMENT PRODUCTS
Some herbs and supplements can be harmful to kidneys.
OTHER MEDICINES
Certain medicines for cancer, blood pressure, heart and other conditions may affect kidneys.
USE MEDICINES SAFELY
CONSULT YOUR DOCTOR
Always consult your doctor before taking any new medicine, including over-the-counter medicines and supplements.
FOLLOW PRESCRIPTION
Take medicines only as prescribed. Do not change the dose or stop without consulting your doctor.
AVOID LONG-TERM USE
Do not use painkillers or other medicines for long periods without medical advice.
KNOW YOUR KIDNEY HEALTH
Get regular kidney check-ups, especially if you have diabetes, high blood pressure or are on long-term medications.
STAY HYDRATED
Drink enough water unless advised otherwise by your doctor.
WATCH FOR SIDE EFFECTS
Report any unusual symptoms like swelling, decreased urine, nausea or fatigue to your doctor.
WHO IS AT HIGHER RISK?
People with diabetes
140 90
People with high blood pressure
People with existing kidney disease
Older adults
People taking multiple medicines
Dehydrated or heavy alcohol users
RIGHT MEDICINE. RIGHT DOSE. RIGHT TIME.
SAFE MEDICINE USE TODAY FOR HEALTHY KIDNEYS TOMORROW.
ALWAYS CHECK. ALWAYS CARE.

Pain Medicines: A Common Risk

One of the most common causes of medication-related kidney problems is the frequent use of certain pain medicines.

Particular caution is needed with:

- Nonsteroidal anti-inflammatory drugs, often called NSAIDs

These medicines can:

- Reduce blood flow to the kidneys
- Worsen kidney function over time

Occasional use may be acceptable for many people, but regular use without guidance can be harmful.

Certain Antibiotics and Medical Agents

Some antibiotics and other medical agents can also affect kidney function.

These include:

- Strong antibiotics used for serious infections
- Contrast dyes used in imaging studies

These treatments are often necessary, but they should be used carefully with proper monitoring.

The Hidden Risk of Over-the-Counter and Herbal Products

Many people believe that medicines available without a prescription, or labeled as “natural,” are always safe.

This is not always true.

Some over-the-counter products and herbal supplements:

- Contain substances that may harm the kidneys
- May interact with prescribed medications

Because these products are not always strictly regulated, their safety can be uncertain.

It is always safer to discuss them with your doctor.

Why Dose Adjustment Matters

As kidney function declines, the way the body handles medicines changes.

Drugs that are normally cleared by the kidneys may:

- Stay longer in the body
- Build up to higher levels
- Cause unwanted effects

That is why doctors often adjust doses based on kidney function.

This is a routine and important part of safe care.

A Practical Example

A patient with mild kidney disease begins taking over-the-counter pain medication regularly for joint discomfort.

Over time:

- Kidney function gradually worsens

After reviewing medications and making adjustments:

- The decline slows

This is a common and preventable situation.

Doctor's Pearl

Every medicine should have a clear purpose. If you are unsure, ask.

Common Mistake to Avoid

Taking over-the-counter medicines regularly without informing your doctor.

Red Flag Warning

Seek medical advice if:

- Kidney function worsens after starting a new medication
- You are using pain medicines frequently
- You are unsure about the safety of a drug or supplement

Key Points

- Some medicines protect kidney function
- Others can harm the kidneys if misused
- Pain medications are a common source of avoidable damage
- Over-the-counter and herbal products are not always safe
- Dose adjustment is important in kidney disease
- Regular medication review is essential

Chapter Summary

Medicines play a central role in kidney care. While certain drugs help control underlying conditions and protect kidney function, others can cause harm if used improperly. The difference lies in correct use, proper dosing, and regular monitoring.

Clear communication with your doctor and careful use of medications can prevent many avoidable problems and support long-term kidney health.

Action Plan

- Take medicines only as prescribed
- Avoid frequent use of pain medications without guidance
- Inform your doctor about all medicines and supplements
- Monitor kidney function regularly
- Ask about dose adjustments if you have kidney disease

Transition to the Next Chapter

As kidney disease progresses, care becomes more complex. In the next chapter, we will discuss advanced kidney disease, what it means, and how to prepare for the next stage of care.

CHAPTER 14: When Kidney Disease Reaches an Advanced Stage

Facing This Stage With Clarity

For some patients, despite careful management, kidney function declines over time and reaches an advanced stage.

Hearing this can be unsettling.

I understand that reaction. Words like "advanced disease" naturally create concern. But I want to approach this differently.

This stage is not just about decline. It is about preparation, planning, and thoughtful care.

When you understand what is happening, you replace fear with clarity and control.

What Changes in the Body

As kidney function becomes significantly reduced, the body begins to struggle to maintain its internal balance.

You may notice:

- Increased fatigue
- Loss of appetite

- Occasional nausea
- Difficulty concentrating
- Changes in sleep

These symptoms develop gradually. They reflect the accumulation of waste products and the reduced ability of the kidneys to maintain balance.

Fluid Retention Becomes More Noticeable

One of the most visible changes in advanced kidney disease is fluid retention.

When the kidneys cannot remove excess fluid effectively:

- Swelling develops in the legs and feet
- Puffiness appears around the eyes
- Body weight may increase

In more serious situations:

- Fluid may collect in the lungs
- Breathing may become uncomfortable

This requires careful management of both fluid intake and medications.

Electrolyte Balance Becomes Critical

The kidneys regulate important minerals in the body.

In advanced disease:

- Potassium levels may rise
- Acid levels may increase
- Sodium balance may fluctuate

These changes may not always produce early symptoms, but they can have serious consequences if not monitored.

Regular blood tests become even more important at this stage.

Blood Pressure Control Becomes More Challenging

As kidney function declines:

- Blood pressure often becomes harder to control
- Medications may need adjustment
- Fluctuations may become more noticeable

This reflects the close relationship between the kidneys and blood pressure.

Managing one helps stabilize the other.

The Emotional Impact

This stage is not only physical.

Patients often experience:

- Anxiety about the future
- Concern about treatment options

- Emotional fatigue

Families may feel the same.

It is important to acknowledge these feelings.

Support from family, healthcare providers, and, when needed, counseling can make a meaningful difference.

The Importance of Planning Ahead

One of the most valuable steps at this stage is planning.

This includes:

- Understanding your current level of kidney function
- Discussing future treatment options
- Preparing for possible dialysis
- Considering transplant options

Planning does not mean that these steps are needed immediately.

It means you are ready, informed, and prepared if they become necessary.

When to Involve a Specialist

At this stage, care from a kidney specialist becomes essential.

You should be under specialist care if:

- Kidney function is significantly reduced
- There is a steady decline over time
- Complications are difficult to manage

A nephrologist can:

- Optimize treatment
- Monitor progression closely
- Guide preparation for advanced therapies

Conservative Care: A Thoughtful Option

Not all patients choose aggressive treatment.

In some situations, especially in older or frail individuals:

- Conservative, supportive care may be appropriate

This approach focuses on:

- Comfort
- Symptom relief
- Quality of life

It is a valid and thoughtful option that should be discussed openly.

KIDNEY DISEASE:
RISK FACTORS, SYMPTOMS & PREVENTION

Kidney disease can affect anyone. Know the risk factors, watch for symptoms and take steps to protect your kidneys.

RISK FACTORS

- **DIABETES** — High blood sugar can damage the kidneys over time.
- **HIGH BLOOD PRESSURE** — High blood pressure can harm blood vessels in kidneys.
- **OBESITY** — Extra weight increases the risk of kidney disease.
- **FAMILY HISTORY** — Kidney disease can run in families.
- **AGE** — Risk increases as you get older.
- **CERTAIN MEDICINES** — Long-term use of painkillers and some medicines can harm kidneys.
- **SMOKING** — Smoking reduces blood flow to kidneys and increases risk.

SYMPTOMS

- **FATIGUE** — Feeling tired or weak most of the time.
- **SWELLING** — Swelling in feet, ankles, legs or face due to fluid buildup.
- **CHANGES IN URINATION** — More or less urine, especially at night, or foamy urine.
- **NAUSEA OR VOMITING** — Waste buildup in the body can cause nausea or loss of appetite.
- **HEADACHE OR POOR FOCUS** — Toxins buildup can cause headaches and trouble focusing.
- **PALE SKIN** — Kidney disease can cause anemia, making skin look pale.
- **LOSS OF APPETITE** — You may not feel like eating or lose weight unintentionally.

Early symptoms may be mild or unnoticed.
Regular check-ups can help detect kidney problems early.

PREVENTION

- **CONTROL BLOOD SUGAR** — Keep diabetes under control.
- **CONTROL BLOOD PRESSURE** — Keep blood pressure in the normal range.
- **DRINK ENOUGH WATER** — Stay hydrated and help your kidneys work better.
- **EAT HEALTHY** — Eat a balanced diet low in salt, sugar and processed foods.
- **STAY ACTIVE** — Exercise regularly and maintain a healthy weight.
- **QUIT SMOKING** — Avoid tobacco to protect your kidneys and overall health.
- **REGULAR CHECK-UPS** — Get kidney tests done if you have risk factors.

Healthy kidneys, healthy life.
Take care today for a better tomorrow.

A Practical Clinical Situation

A patient with long-standing kidney disease begins to feel more tired.

Swelling develops in the legs.

Tests show further decline in kidney function.

At this stage:

- Medications are adjusted
- Diet is modified
- A specialist is involved

With proper planning, the patient is prepared for future decisions without panic.

Doctor's Pearl

Advanced kidney disease is a stage for preparation, not panic.

Common Mistake to Avoid

Delaying specialist care until symptoms become severe.

Red Flag Warning

Seek urgent care if you experience:

- Severe shortness of breath
- Persistent vomiting
- Confusion
- Rapidly increasing swelling

Key Points

- Advanced kidney disease involves significant loss of function
- Symptoms become more noticeable
- Fluid and electrolyte balance become difficult
- Emotional impact is important
- Planning ahead improves outcomes
- Specialist care is essential

Chapter Summary

Advanced kidney disease represents a stage where the kidneys can no longer maintain balance effectively. Symptoms become more noticeable, and complications require careful management. At the same time, this stage provides an opportunity to plan ahead and make informed decisions.

With proper medical care, emotional support, and thoughtful preparation, this phase can be managed in a structured and less stressful way.

Action Plan

- Understand your current stage of kidney disease
- Follow medical advice closely
- Monitor symptoms and report changes
- Discuss future treatment options early
- Stay connected with your healthcare team

Transition to the Next Chapter

As kidney disease progresses further, some patients may require dialysis or kidney transplantation. In the next chapter, we will discuss these options in a clear and practical way so you know what to expect and how to prepare.

CHAPTER 15: Dialysis and Kidney Transplant: Knowing Your Options

When the Kidneys Need Support

There may come a stage when the kidneys are no longer able to maintain the body's internal balance.

At this point:

- Waste products begin to build up
- Fluid cannot be removed effectively
- Electrolytes become unstable

This stage is often called **kidney failure** or **end-stage kidney disease**.

When this happens, the body needs support.

That support comes in two main forms:

- Dialysis
- Kidney transplantation

These words can sound intimidating, but understanding them clearly makes them far less frightening.

Dialysis: Supporting the Body

Dialysis is a treatment that performs some of the functions of the kidneys.

It helps:

- Remove waste products from the blood
- Remove excess fluid
- Maintain mineral balance

It does not replace all kidney functions, but it can keep the body stable and allow patients to continue their daily lives.

Hemodialysis: The Most Common Form

In hemodialysis:

- Blood is taken from the body
- Passed through a machine that filters it
- Returned to the body

This is usually done:

- At a dialysis center
- About three times a week
- Each session lasting several hours

At first, this routine may feel overwhelming.

With time, many patients adapt and organize their lives around it.

Peritoneal Dialysis: A Home-Based Option

Peritoneal dialysis offers more flexibility.

In this method:

- A special fluid is placed into the abdomen
- The lining of the abdomen acts as a natural filter
- Waste products move into this fluid
- The fluid is then drained

This can often be done:

- At home
- During the day or overnight

It requires training and discipline, but it gives more independence.

Living With Dialysis

Starting dialysis is a significant change.

There may be:

- Adjustments in daily routine
- Changes in diet and fluid intake
- Regular medical visits

At the same time, it is important to understand:

Many patients:

- Continue working

- Spend time with family
- Remain active

With proper support and planning, life continues in a meaningful way.

Kidney Transplant: A Different Approach

A kidney transplant involves placing a healthy kidney from a donor into the body.

The donor may be:

- A living donor
- A deceased donor

A successful transplant can:

- Restore near-normal kidney function
- Improve energy and quality of life
- Provide greater freedom compared to dialysis

For many patients, this is the preferred long-term option.

Life After Transplant

After a transplant:

- Patients often feel stronger and more energetic
- Dietary restrictions are usually less strict

However, it requires ongoing care.

Patients must:

- Take medications regularly to prevent rejection
- Monitor for infections
- Attend regular follow-up visits

With proper care, many patients do very well for years.

Choosing the Right Option

There is no single answer for everyone.

The decision depends on:

- Overall health
- Age
- Availability of a donor
- Personal preference
- Lifestyle considerations

Some patients begin with dialysis and later receive a transplant.

The most important step is understanding your options and making an informed decision.

Emotional Aspects

Facing kidney failure is not only a medical challenge.

It is also emotional.

Patients may feel:

- Fear
- Uncertainty
- Anxiety about the future

Families may feel the same.

It is important to acknowledge these feelings and seek support when needed.

You are not alone in this journey.

A Practical Example

A patient with advanced kidney disease prepares early.

He:

- Learns about dialysis
- Visits a dialysis center
- Discusses transplant options

When treatment becomes necessary:

- Dialysis begins smoothly
- Adjustment is easier

Preparation makes a real difference.

KIDNEY CARE OPTIONS

DIALYSIS AND TRANSPLANT

When kidneys can no longer work well

If your kidneys fail and cannot clean your blood, treatment can help you live a longer and healthier life.

DIALYSIS

A treatment that removes waste, excess fluid and toxins from your blood when your kidneys can no longer do it.

HEMODIALYSIS

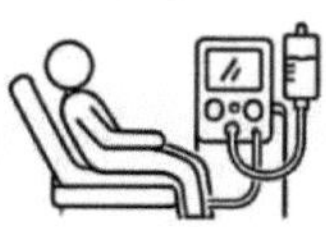

- Blood is filtered through a machine.
- Usually done 3 times a week.
- Takes about 3–5 hours each session.

PERITONEAL DIALYSIS

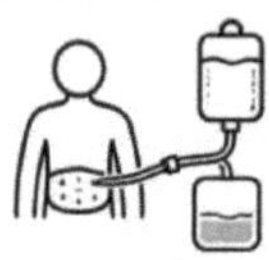

- The lining of your abdomen filters your blood.
- Can be done at home.
- Done daily.

KIDNEY TRANSPLANT

A surgery to receive a healthy kidney from a donor. It can be from a living or deceased donor.

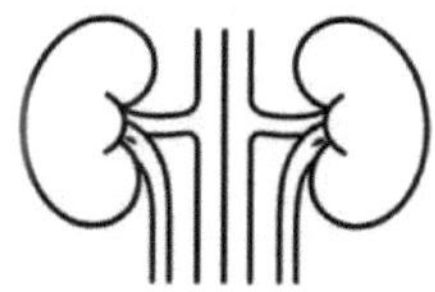

- Best option for many people with kidney failure.
- Better quality of life and longer life expectancy.
- Requires surgery and lifelong medicines to prevent rejection.
- A living donor can be a family member or a friend.

COMPARISON

FEATURE	DIALYSIS	KIDNEY TRANSPLANT
Treatment	Ongoing treatment	One-time surgery
Time Commitment	Regular sessions (multiple times a week or daily)	Recovery time after surgery, then regular follow-up
Quality of Life	Good, but with some restrictions	Better quality of life for most people
Medicines	Some medicines	Lifelong medicines to prevent rejecton
Cost	Ongoing cost	High initially, then ongoing medication cost

IMPORTANT REMINDERS

- Follow your doctor's advice and treatment plan.
- Take medicines as prescribed.
- Eat a kidney-friendly diet and limit salt.
- Stay active as advised by your doctor.
- Seek support from family, friends and support groups.

EARLY CARE, RIGHT TREATMENT, BETTER LIFE.

Your choice, your health, your future.

Doctor's Pearl

Early preparation makes the transition to dialysis or transplant much smoother.

Common Mistake to Avoid

Waiting until the last moment to learn about treatment options.

Red Flag Warning

Seek urgent care if you experience:

- Severe breathlessness
- Persistent vomiting
- Confusion
- Very low urine output

Key Points

- Dialysis and transplant are life-saving treatments
- Hemodialysis and peritoneal dialysis are the main types
- Transplant offers better long-term quality of life for many patients
- Early preparation is essential
- Emotional support is important

Chapter Summary

When kidney function declines to a critical level, dialysis or transplantation becomes necessary. Dialysis supports the body by removing waste and excess fluid, while transplantation offers a more long-term solution by restoring kidney function.

Understanding these options in advance helps patients make informed decisions and approach the future with confidence.

Action Plan

- Discuss dialysis options early with your doctor
- Learn about transplant possibilities
- Prepare mentally and practically
- Involve your family in planning
- Maintain regular follow-up

Transition to the Next Chapter

Now that we have discussed advanced kidney disease and its treatment, let us turn to a very common condition that affects many people. In the next chapter, we will discuss kidney stones, why they form, and how they can be prevented.

CHAPTER 16: Kidney Stones: Why They Form and Why They Return

A Common Problem That Deserves Better Understanding

Kidney stones are one of the most common causes of sudden, severe pain.

Many patients remember the experience very clearly. The pain is intense, unexpected, and often frightening. After the episode passes, life returns to normal, and the problem is often forgotten.

But that is where the real issue begins.

Kidney stones are not just an isolated event. They are often a recurring condition.

Unless you understand why they form, there is a strong chance they will return.

What Exactly Is a Kidney Stone

A kidney stone is a hard deposit made from minerals and salts in the urine.

Under normal conditions:

- These substances remain dissolved

- They pass out of the body without difficulty

When the balance changes:

- Urine becomes concentrated
- Crystals begin to form
- These crystals join together and grow

Over time, these crystals form a stone.

The stone may:

- Stay in the kidney without causing symptoms
- Move into the urinary tract
- Cause severe pain when it blocks urine flow

The Basic Mechanism: Concentration and Imbalance

At its core, stone formation is simple.

It happens when:

- Urine is too concentrated
- Stone-forming substances are too high
- Protective substances are too low

In practical terms:

The less diluted your urine, the higher the risk of stone formation.

This is why hydration plays such an important role.

KIDNEY STONES

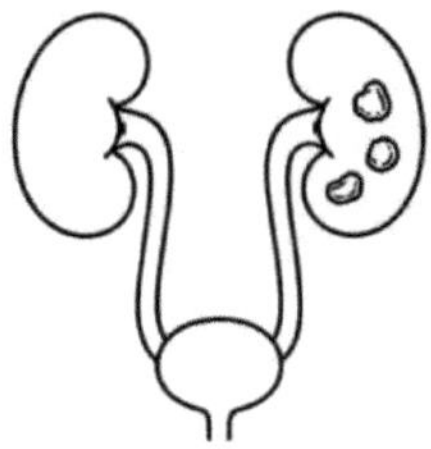

Hard deposits made of minerals and salts that form in the kidneys. They can cause severe pain if not treated.

COMMON SYMPTOMS

- Severe pain in back, side or lower abdomen
- Pain or burning during urination
- Bloody or cloudy urine
- Nausea or vomiting
- Needing to urinate more often

COMMON CAUSES

- Not drinking enough water
- High salt intake
- High animal protein intake
- Obesity
- Family history of kidney stones

PREVENTION

- **Drink plenty of water** (2.5–3 liters daily)
- **Eat less salt** (less than 5 grams daily)
- **Eat a balanced diet** more fruits, vegetables and whole grains
- **Maintain a healthy weight**
- **Limit sugary drinks and alcohol**

TREATMENT OPTIONS

Treatment depends on the size of the stone and your symptoms.

Medication
Pain relievers and medicines help pass small stones.

Drink more fluids
Helps flush out small stones naturally.

Shock Wave Lithotripsy (ESWL)
High-energy waves break stones into small pieces that pass in urine.

Ureteroscopy
A thin scope is used to remove or break stones.

SEE A DOCTOR IF YOU HAVE:

- Severe pain that does not get better
- Fever or chills
- Blood in urine
- Persistent vomiting
- Pain lasting more than a few days

Types of Kidney Stones

Not all stones are the same. Understanding the type helps guide prevention.

Calcium Stones

- The most common type
- Often related to calcium and oxalate levels

Uric Acid Stones

- Form in more acidic urine
- More common in people with high uric acid

Struvite Stones

- Associated with infections
- Can grow quickly

Cystine Stones

- Rare
- Usually due to genetic conditions

Each type has a different underlying cause, which is why proper evaluation is important after a stone episode.

Everyday Risk Factors

Several common factors increase the risk of kidney stones.

These include:

- Low fluid intake
- High salt intake
- Diets high in certain substances such as oxalate
- Obesity
- Sedentary lifestyle
- Family history

Climate also plays a role.

In hot weather:

- Increased sweating leads to dehydration
- Urine becomes more concentrated

This increases the risk of stone formation.

Why Stones Come Back

One of the most frustrating aspects of kidney stones is recurrence.

Many patients experience repeated episodes.

This usually happens because:

- The underlying cause remains unchanged
- Hydration habits are not improved
- Diet is not adjusted

Without addressing these factors, the same process continues.

How Stones Grow Over Time

Stone formation is usually gradual.

It begins with:

- Tiny crystals in the urine

These:

- Join together
- Slowly increase in size

Small stones may pass unnoticed.

Larger stones are more likely to cause symptoms when they move or block urine flow.

A Familiar Clinical Pattern

A patient experiences severe pain and is diagnosed with a kidney stone.

The stone passes or is treated.

Symptoms improve.

No further evaluation is done.

After some time:

- Another episode occurs

This pattern repeats.

The reason is simple.

The cause was never addressed.

Doctor's Pearl

Kidney stones are often preventable. Understanding the cause is the key.

Common Mistake to Avoid

Ignoring a stone episode once the pain resolves.

Red Flag Warning

Seek immediate care if you have:

- Severe, persistent pain
- Fever with urinary symptoms
- Blood in urine
- Difficulty passing urine

Key Points

- Kidney stones form from crystallization of minerals in urine
- Concentrated urine increases risk

- There are different types of stones with different causes
- Recurrence is common if causes are not addressed
- Prevention is possible

Chapter Summary

Kidney stones are a common and often painful condition. They develop when minerals and salts in the urine become concentrated and form crystals that grow into stones. A variety of factors, including low fluid intake, diet, and metabolic tendencies, contribute to their formation.

The most important aspect of kidney stones is their tendency to recur. Without addressing the underlying causes, many patients experience repeated episodes. The good news is that with proper understanding and preventive measures, the risk can be significantly reduced.

Action Plan

- Increase daily fluid intake
- Reduce excess salt in your diet
- Maintain a healthy weight
- Be mindful of dietary risk factors
- Seek evaluation after even one stone episode

Transition to the Next Chapter

Now that you understand how kidney stones form, the next step is to recognize how they present and how they are treated. In the next chapter, we will discuss symptoms, diagnosis, and treatment in a clear and practical way.

CHAPTER 17: Kidney Stones: Symptoms, Diagnosis, and Treatment

When a Stone Makes Itself Known

Unlike many kidney conditions that stay silent for years, kidney stones often announce themselves suddenly and forcefully.

The most common symptom is pain, and it is not mild.

Patients often describe it as:

- Sudden in onset
- Severe and sharp
- Coming in waves
- Difficult to tolerate

This type of pain is called **renal colic**.

It usually begins in the side or back and may travel:

- Toward the lower abdomen
- Into the groin

One important feature is restlessness.

Patients often move around, unable to find a comfortable position. This is different from many other types of pain where lying still provides relief.

Other Symptoms That May Occur

Pain is the main symptom, but it is often accompanied by other signs.

These may include:

- Blood in the urine, making it appear pink or red
- Nausea and vomiting
- Burning during urination
- Frequent urge to pass urine

If infection is present, additional symptoms may appear:

- Fever
- Chills

This combination requires urgent attention.

When It Becomes an Emergency

Not every kidney stone requires emergency care, but certain situations should never be ignored.

Seek immediate medical attention if there is:

- Fever with urinary symptoms
- Severe pain not controlled by medication
- Persistent vomiting
- Inability to pass urine

These may indicate:

- Infection

- Complete obstruction
- Risk of kidney damage

Prompt treatment is essential.

How the Diagnosis Is Made

Diagnosis is based on symptoms and tests.

Urine Tests

- Detect blood, infection, or crystals

Blood Tests

- Evaluate kidney function
- Check electrolyte levels

Imaging Studies

- CT scan is the most accurate
- Ultrasound is often used as an initial test

These tests help determine:

- Presence of a stone
- Size and location
- Any complications

When Stones Pass Naturally

Many stones, especially small ones, pass on their own.

In such cases, treatment focuses on:

- Pain relief
- Adequate hydration
- Medications that help relax the urinary tract

Patients are usually advised to:

- Drink fluids
- Stay active
- Monitor urine

Passage may take time, but many stones resolve without procedures.

When Treatment Is Needed

Not all stones pass on their own.

Larger stones or complicated cases may require intervention.

Common options include:

Shock Wave Therapy

- Breaks stones into smaller pieces

Endoscopic Procedures

- Use small instruments to remove or break stones

Surgery

- Reserved for large or complex stones

The choice depends on:

- Size of the stone
- Location
- Severity of symptoms
- Overall health

Recovery and Follow-Up

Once the stone passes or is treated:

- Symptoms usually improve quickly

But treatment does not end there.

Follow-up is important to:

- Confirm that the stone has cleared
- Identify the type of stone
- Evaluate risk factors

This helps prevent recurrence.

Prevention: The Most Important Step

The most important part of management is prevention.

This includes:

- Adequate hydration

- Reducing salt intake
- Adjusting diet based on stone type
- Maintaining a healthy weight
- Using medications when needed

Consistency is essential.

A Practical Example

A patient presents with severe flank pain and is diagnosed with a small kidney stone.

With pain control and hydration:

- The stone passes

Later, he improves his habits:

- Drinks more fluids
- Reduces salt intake

He remains free from recurrence.

This is the goal of treatment.

Doctor's Pearl

Relieving pain is only the first step. Preventing recurrence is the real success.

Common Mistake to Avoid

Stopping care after the first stone episode.

Red Flag Warning

Seek urgent care if you experience:

- Fever with urinary symptoms
- Severe uncontrolled pain
- Persistent vomiting
- Reduced urine output

Key Points

- Kidney stones often cause severe, wave-like pain
- Blood in urine and nausea are common
- Small stones may pass naturally
- Larger stones may require procedures
- Diagnosis depends on tests and imaging
- Prevention is essential

Chapter Summary

Kidney stones are a common cause of severe pain. While many stones pass on their own, others require medical or surgical treatment. Diagnosis is based on symptoms and imaging, and treatment depends on the size and location of the stone.

The most important aspect of care is prevention. With proper hydration, dietary changes, and medical guidance, the risk of recurrence can be significantly reduced.

Action Plan

- Increase daily fluid intake
- Seek care promptly for severe symptoms
- Follow up after a stone episode
- Adjust diet as advised
- Maintain preventive habits

Transition to the Next Chapter

Now that you understand kidney stones in detail, the next step is to clear common doubts. In the next chapter, we will address myths and frequently asked questions so you can make informed decisions with confidence.

CHAPTER 18: Myths, Misconceptions, and Questions Patients Often Ask

Why Confusion Is So Common

Kidney disease is common, but clear understanding is not.

Patients often receive advice from many sources:

- Friends and family
- Internet searches
- Social media
- Personal experiences of others

Some of this information is helpful. Much of it is incomplete or misleading.

Over time, this creates confusion, unnecessary fear, and sometimes wrong decisions.

This chapter is meant to bring clarity.

Myth: "If I Feel Fine, My Kidneys Must Be Fine"

Reality

This is one of the most common and most dangerous assumptions.

Early kidney disease often has no symptoms.

You may feel completely normal while:

- Kidney function is slowly declining
- Protein is leaking into the urine

This is why regular testing is essential.

Myth: "A Slightly Abnormal Creatinine Means Serious Disease"

Reality

A single abnormal number does not tell the full story.

What matters is:

- The trend over time
- The eGFR
- The overall clinical picture

Many patients have mildly abnormal values that remain stable for years.

The key is proper interpretation, not panic.

Myth: "Drinking More Water Will Cure Kidney Disease"

Reality

Water is important, but it is not a cure.

Adequate hydration:

- Supports kidney function
- Helps prevent kidney stones

But:

- It does not reverse established kidney disease
- Excessive intake may not always help

Balance is important.

Myth: "I Should Avoid All Protein"

Reality

Protein is essential for the body.

Very high protein intake may increase the workload on the kidneys, but complete avoidance is not healthy.

Too little protein can lead to:

- Weakness
- Loss of muscle
- Poor overall health

Moderation is the right approach.

Myth: “Natural or Herbal Products Are Always Safe”

Reality

Natural does not always mean safe.

Some herbal products:

- May harm the kidneys
- May interact with medications

Because these products are not always well regulated, their safety can be uncertain.

Always discuss them with your doctor.

Myth: “Kidney Stones Are a One-Time Problem”

Reality

Kidney stones often recur.

If underlying causes are not addressed:

- Stones may form again

Prevention is essential.

Frequently Asked Questions

Let me address some common questions.

How often should I check my kidney function?
It depends on your risk. If you have diabetes or high blood pressure, regular testing is important.

Can kidney disease be reversed?
In many cases, it cannot be fully reversed, but progression can often be slowed.

Is dialysis always permanent?
In chronic kidney disease, it is usually long term unless a transplant is done. In acute kidney injury, it may be temporary.

Can I live a normal life with kidney disease?
Yes. With proper care, many patients lead active and fulfilling lives.

Diet Confusion: What Really Matters

Patients often receive conflicting dietary advice.

The truth is simpler.

- Extreme diets are rarely necessary
- Balance is more important than restriction
- Salt control is essential
- Hydration should be appropriate

Consistency matters more than complexity.

Water Intake: A Common Question

"How much water should I drink?"

There is no single answer for everyone.

- Healthy individuals benefit from adequate hydration
- Kidney stone patients may need more fluids
- Advanced kidney disease may require fluid restriction

Individualization is key.

A Real-Life Example

A patient reads online that drinking excessive amounts of water can cure kidney disease.

He begins consuming large volumes daily.

Soon:

- He develops swelling
- Electrolyte balance is affected

This shows how incorrect information can lead to harm.

Doctor's Pearl

Correct understanding leads to correct decisions.

Common Mistake to Avoid

Following advice from unreliable sources.

Red Flag Warning

Be cautious if:

- You are trying unproven remedies
- You are making extreme dietary changes
- You are ignoring medical advice

Key Points

- Many myths exist about kidney disease
- Early disease may have no symptoms
- Lab results must be interpreted properly
- Hydration helps but is not a cure
- Balanced diet is essential
- Prevention is important in kidney stones

Chapter Summary

Kidney disease is often surrounded by misconceptions that lead to confusion and poor decisions. By understanding the facts, patients can avoid unnecessary fear and focus on practical steps that truly protect their health.

Reliable information is one of the most powerful tools in managing kidney disease.

Action Plan

- Rely on evidence-based information
- Discuss doubts with your doctor
- Avoid extreme or unverified health practices
- Follow a balanced diet and hydration plan
- Stay consistent with monitoring and care

Transition to the Next Chapter

You now have a clear understanding of kidney health and disease. In the final chapter, we will bring everything together into a simple, practical plan you can follow for life.

CHAPTER 19: A Lifetime Plan to Protect Your Kidneys

Bringing Everything Together

You have now come to the final chapter of this book.

We have discussed how the kidneys work, how disease begins, how it progresses, how it affects the body, and how it can be treated.

But information alone is not enough.

What matters now is what you do with it.

Kidney health is not built in a day. It is built over years through small, consistent choices.

This chapter is about turning understanding into action.

Think Simple, Not Complicated

Many people look for a detailed plan or a perfect routine.

You do not need that.

Kidney health rests on a few clear principles:

- Awareness
- Regular monitoring
- Control of risk factors
- Healthy daily habits

- Proper use of medications

These are simple ideas, but they are powerful when practiced consistently.

Start With Awareness

The first step is awareness.

Know your risk:

- Do you have diabetes?
- High blood pressure?
- A history of kidney stones?
- A family history of kidney disease?

Know your numbers:

- Creatinine
- eGFR
- Urine protein

When you understand your starting point, you are in control.

Focus on What You Can Control

It is easy to feel overwhelmed by disease.

But you do not need to control everything.

You need to focus on what you can control:

- Blood pressure
- Blood sugar
- Diet
- Physical activity
- Weight
- Medication use

These are not small factors. They are the main drivers of long-term outcomes.

Small Steps, Big Results

You do not need dramatic changes.

Small, steady steps are more effective.

For example:

- Reducing salt in your meals
- Walking regularly
- Drinking adequate fluids
- Taking medicines consistently

These habits may seem simple, but over time, they make a significant difference.

Consistency Matters More Than Perfection

Many people begin with strong motivation and try to change everything at once.

That approach often does not last.

You do not need perfection.

You need consistency.

Even modest improvements, maintained over time, protect your kidneys.

Stay Connected With Your Doctor

Kidney health is not something you manage alone.

Regular follow-up helps to:

- Monitor kidney function
- Adjust treatment when needed
- Detect problems early

Do not hesitate to ask questions.

Understanding your condition gives you confidence.

Listen to Your Body

Your body often gives early signals.

Pay attention to:

- Changes in urination
- Swelling
- Fatigue
- Blood pressure changes

These signs may be subtle, but they are important.

Do Not Ignore Kidney Stones

If you have had kidney stones:

- Prevention should become part of your routine

This includes:

- Adequate hydration
- Dietary awareness
- Follow-up when needed

Even one episode is important.

A Practical Long-Term Plan

Let us bring everything together.

- Get regular blood and urine tests
- Control blood pressure and blood sugar
- Eat a balanced, low-salt diet
- Stay physically active
- Avoid unnecessary medications
- Stay well hydrated
- Follow medical advice consistently

This is not complicated.

But it requires commitment.

A Reflection From Practice

Over the years, I have seen two different patterns.

Some patients ignore early signs and delay care. Over time, they face more serious problems.

Others take early advice seriously:

- They make small, steady changes
- They stay engaged in their care
- They follow up regularly

The difference in outcomes is clear.

Doctor's Pearl

Kidney health is protected by consistent daily habits, not occasional effort.

Common Mistake to Avoid

Waiting for symptoms before taking action.

Red Flag Warning

Do not ignore:

- Rising blood pressure
- Persistent swelling
- Changes in urination
- Unexplained fatigue

Key Points

- Kidney health requires long-term attention
- Many risk factors are controllable
- Small steps lead to meaningful results
- Consistency is more important than intensity
- Regular monitoring improves outcomes

Chapter Summary

Protecting your kidneys is a lifelong process built on awareness, consistency, and informed choices. Kidney disease can be serious, but it is often manageable, especially when detected early and treated properly.

Simple habits, followed consistently, can preserve kidney function and maintain quality of life for many years.

Action Plan

- Schedule regular kidney function tests
- Monitor blood pressure and blood sugar
- Follow a balanced, low-salt diet
- Stay physically active

- Use medications responsibly
- Stay engaged in your care

Final Message

Your kidneys work quietly for you every day.

Take care of them with the same quiet consistency.

The effort you make today will protect your health for years to come.

APPENDIX 1: Understanding Your Kidney Tests in a Simple Way

Do Not Let the Numbers Intimidate You

Many patients feel uneasy when they first look at their lab reports.

The terms seem technical. The numbers appear confusing. A small change can create unnecessary worry.

Let me reassure you.

Your lab report is not meant to frighten you. It is meant to guide you.

Once you understand a few key points, these numbers become clear and useful.

Creatinine: A Starting Point

Creatinine is a waste product from normal muscle activity.

Healthy kidneys remove it from the blood.

When kidney function declines:

- Creatinine rises

This seems simple, but there is an important detail.

Creatinine varies from person to person.

It depends on:

- Age
- Body size
- Muscle mass

A muscular individual may naturally have a higher creatinine than someone smaller or older.

So this number must always be interpreted in context.

---

eGFR: A Better Indicator

To better understand kidney function, we use **eGFR**, or estimated glomerular filtration rate.

It is calculated from creatinine along with age and other factors.

In simple terms:

- Higher eGFR means better kidney function
- Lower eGFR indicates reduced function

A general idea helps:

- Above 90 is usually normal
- 60 to 89 suggests mild reduction
- 30 to 59 indicates moderate reduction
- Below 30 reflects more significant loss

But the most important point is this:

The trend over time matters more than a single value.

Protein in Urine: An Early Warning

Healthy kidneys prevent protein from leaking into urine.

When the filters are affected:

- Protein appears in the urine

This is often one of the earliest signs of kidney damage.

It may not cause symptoms, which is why testing is important.

Even small amounts can be significant.

Urine Test: Simple but Valuable

A routine urine test can provide important information.

It can detect:

- Protein
- Blood
- Infection
- Crystals

This simple test often gives the first clue to a problem.

Electrolytes: Internal Balance

Kidneys help maintain the balance of important minerals.

These include:

- Potassium
- Sodium
- Bicarbonate

When kidney function declines:

- These levels may become abnormal

This can affect:

- Heart rhythm
- Muscle function
- Overall stability

Hemoglobin: Why Anemia Occurs

The kidneys produce a hormone that supports red blood cell production.

When kidney function declines:

- Hemoglobin levels may fall

This leads to anemia.

Patients may feel:

- Tired
- Weak
- Less energetic

How to Read Your Report

When reviewing your lab results:

- Do not focus on a single number
- Compare with previous reports
- Look for trends
- Discuss findings with your doctor

This approach provides clarity and avoids unnecessary worry.

Doctor's Pearl

Your lab report tells a story. Understand it over time, not in a single reading.

Key Points

- Creatinine is useful but must be interpreted in context
- eGFR gives a clearer picture of kidney function
- Protein in urine is an early warning sign
- Urine tests can detect problems early
- Electrolytes reflect internal balance
- Hemoglobin helps identify anemia

Summary

Kidney tests are simple but powerful tools. When understood properly, they help detect problems early, monitor progress, and guide treatment. Instead of causing anxiety, they should give you clarity and confidence in managing your health.

Transition to Next Appendix

Now that you understand your test reports, the next step is practical.

In the next appendix, we will look at a simple, kidney-friendly diet that you can follow comfortably every day.

APPENDIX 2: A Simple and Practical Kidney-Friendly Diet Guide

Let Us Simplify Diet

Diet is one of the most confusing areas for patients.

Many people are told to avoid too many things. Others follow strict plans for a few weeks and then give up. Some feel that eating for kidney health is too complicated to maintain.

It does not have to be that way.

A good diet is not complicated.
It is simple, balanced, and consistent.

That is what protects your kidneys over time.

The Basic Principle

A kidney-friendly diet is not about severe restriction.

It is about:

- Balance
- Moderation
- Consistency

The goal is to:

- Support overall health
- Control blood pressure and blood sugar
- Reduce stress on the kidneys

If you follow these principles, you are already doing the right thing.

What to Include Regularly

Focus on foods that support long-term health.

These include:

- Fresh vegetables
- Fruits in moderate portions
- Whole grains such as oats or brown rice
- Balanced protein sources
- Healthy fats such as olive oil

These foods provide:

- Essential nutrients
- Fiber
- Sustained energy

Keep meals simple and home-cooked whenever possible.

What to Limit

Certain foods increase the burden on the kidneys when taken in excess.

Limit:

- Processed and packaged foods
- Restaurant meals high in salt
- Fried and heavily seasoned foods
- Sugary drinks and excess sweets
- Very high-protein diets

You do not need to eliminate everything.

You need to reduce excess.

Salt: The Most Important Change

If you make only one dietary change, make it this:

Reduce salt intake.

Excess salt:

- Raises blood pressure
- Causes fluid retention
- Increases stress on the kidneys

Most salt comes from:

- Packaged foods
- Snacks
- Pickles and sauces
- Restaurant meals

Simple steps:

- Cook more meals at home

- Avoid adding extra salt at the table
- Read labels when possible

Even small reductions can make a meaningful difference.

Protein: Balanced Intake

Protein is essential, but too much can increase kidney workload.

The goal is balance.

Choose:

- Moderate portions
- A mix of plant and animal sources

Avoid:

- Very high-protein diets unless medically advised

This approach supports both kidney and overall health.

Fluids: Practical Guidance

Fluid intake is a common concern.

For most people:

- Drink enough to stay well hydrated
- Aim for light-colored urine

But remember:

- More is not always better
- Excess fluid does not improve kidney function

In advanced kidney disease:

- Fluid intake may need to be limited

Always follow medical advice when applicable.

Special Considerations

As kidney disease progresses, diet may need adjustment.

This may include monitoring:

- Potassium
- Phosphorus
- Fluid intake

At this stage:

- Diet becomes more individualized
- Medical guidance is important

Do not make major dietary restrictions without advice.

Diet and Kidney Stones

If you have had kidney stones, diet becomes even more important.

Helpful steps:

- Increase fluid intake
- Reduce salt
- Adjust diet based on stone type
- Maintain balanced calcium intake

These changes reduce recurrence.

A Simple Daily Example

A practical approach may look like this:

Breakfast:

- Oatmeal with fruit

Lunch:

- Whole grain with vegetables and moderate protein

Dinner:

- Light meal with vegetables and protein

Snacks:

- Fruits or small portions of nuts

Keep it simple and consistent.

Doctor's Pearl

A simple diet followed consistently is more effective than a strict diet followed briefly.

Common Mistake to Avoid

Following extreme diets that are difficult to maintain.

Red Flag Warning

Consult your doctor before major dietary changes if:

- You have advanced kidney disease
- You have abnormal potassium levels
- You are on fluid restriction

Key Points

- Diet plays a major role in kidney health
- Fresh, simple foods are best
- Reducing salt is essential
- Protein intake should be moderate
- Hydration should be appropriate
- Diet may need adjustment in advanced disease

Summary

A kidney-friendly diet is not about complicated rules. It is about simple, balanced choices made consistently. By focusing on fresh foods, reducing salt, maintaining proper hydration, and avoiding excess, you can protect your kidneys and improve overall health.

Transition to Next Appendix

Now that you understand what to eat, the next step is to put it into action.

In the next appendix, we will create a simple 30-day plan to help you build lasting habits for kidney health.

APPENDIX 3: A Simple 30-Day Plan to Build Lifelong Kidney Health Habits

Turning Knowledge Into Daily Action

By now, you understand kidney health clearly.

You know what affects it, what protects it, and what harms it.

But understanding alone is not enough.

Real benefit comes when knowledge becomes daily action.

That is exactly what this 30-day plan is designed to do.

It is simple, practical, and realistic. It is not meant to be perfect. It is meant to be sustainable.

How to Use This Plan

Keep it simple.

- Focus on one week at a time
- Do not try to change everything at once
- Repeat small actions daily
- If you miss a day, continue without guilt

By the end of 30 days, these steps will begin to feel natural.

WEEK 1: Awareness and Baseline

Focus: Understand Your Starting Point

Before making changes, you need clarity.

Steps for the Week

- Check your blood pressure
- Review or obtain basic blood tests
- Do a urine test if not done recently
- List all your current medications

Daily Habits

- Drink adequate water
- Reduce obvious excess salt

Goal

- Understand where you stand

This is your baseline.

WEEK 2: Improve Diet and Hydration

Focus: Build Better Eating Habits

Now begin simple changes in what you eat and drink.

Steps for the Week

- Reduce salt in cooking
- Avoid processed foods
- Add more vegetables and fruits
- Keep protein intake balanced

Daily Habits

- Eat simple, home-cooked meals
- Stay consistently hydrated

Goal

- Create a balanced, sustainable diet

WEEK 3: Activity and Risk Control

Focus: Strengthen the Body

This week focuses on movement and control of key health factors.

Steps for the Week

- Monitor blood pressure regularly
- Check blood sugar if applicable
- Start a regular activity routine

Daily Habits

- Walk for 20 to 30 minutes
- Stay active throughout the day

Goal

- Improve energy and overall control

WEEK 4: Consistency and Routine

Focus: Make It a Habit

Now bring everything together.

Steps for the Week

- Review medications with your doctor if needed
- Avoid unnecessary over-the-counter medicines
- Plan regular follow-up

Daily Habits

- Take medications consistently
- Maintain diet and activity patterns

Goal

- Build a routine that lasts

At the End of 30 Days

You will notice:

- Better awareness of your health
- Improved daily habits
- More consistency
- Greater confidence in managing your health

This is not the end of a plan.

It is the beginning of a lifestyle.

A Real-Life Perspective

I have seen patients follow simple plans like this.

At first, the changes feel small.

But over time:

- Blood pressure improves
- Blood sugar stabilizes
- Weight becomes easier to manage
- Kidney function remains stable

This is how long-term health is built.

Doctor's Pearl

Small steps repeated daily create lasting health.

Common Mistake to Avoid

Trying to change everything at once and giving up.

Red Flag Warning

Seek medical advice if:

- You feel unwell during changes
- Blood pressure or sugar becomes unstable
- New symptoms appear

Key Points

- A simple plan makes change easier
- Small steps lead to lasting habits
- Consistency is more important than intensity
- Monitoring supports progress
- Lifestyle changes have long-term impact

Summary

This 30-day plan helps you move from understanding to action. By focusing on awareness, diet, activity, and consistency, you build habits that protect your kidneys and improve overall health.

The real success is not completing 30 days.

The real success is continuing these habits for life.

Final Closing Message

Start today.

Keep it simple.

Stay consistent.

Your kidneys work quietly for you every day.

Take care of them with the same quiet consistency.

Thank You and Please Review the Book

Thank you for taking the time to read this book. I sincerely hope it has helped you understand your health a little more clearly and has given you practical, everyday steps you can follow with confidence. If you found this book helpful, **I would truly appreciate it if you could leave a brief and honest review.** Even a few lines sharing your experience can make a meaningful difference. Your feedback helps other readers find reliable, trustworthy health information and supports them in making better decisions for themselves and their families.

Warm regards,

Dr Prabhat Das

Continue your Healthcare Journey with these Books

Good health is a journey, not a single step. It is not achieved in one day or with one book. That is why I created the "Better Health with Dr Das Series", with each book addressing a different common condition. If you would like easy, practical guidance on other everyday health concerns, you may wish to explore the rest of books in this series.

Books in this series:

- Better Health starts Here: A Doctor's Guide to Staying Healthy After 40
- A Doctor's Easy Guide to Understanding & Managing OBESITY
- Doctor, What DIET Is Best for Me?
- Doctor, Why Can't I Lose Weight? A Doctor's Guide to Safe & Sustainable Weight Loss)
- A Doctor's Easy Guide to GLP-1 for Obesity
- A Doctor's Easy Guide to Understanding & Managing HIGH BLOOD PRESSURE
- A Doctor's Guide to Living Well With DIABETES
- A Doctor's Guide to Understanding & Managing THYROID DISEASES
- A Doctor's Guide to Understanding & Managing HIGH CHOLESTEROL
- A Doctor's Practical Guide to HEART HEALTH After 40: How to Protect Your Heart & Live Longer
- A Doctor's Guide to Healing & Reversing FATTY LIVER DISEASE: Simple, Natural & Science-Based Steps to Reduce Liver Fat and Prevent Complications

- Control Your ACID REFLUX, HEARTBURN & GERD: A Doctor's Practical Guide that Works
- Live Comfortably with IRRITABLE BOWEL SYNDROME: A Doctor's Practical Guide to Understanding & Managing IBS
- A Doctor's Practical Guide to Understanding & Managing GALLBLADDER STONES & OTHER PROBLEMS
- Take Control of COPD: A Doctor's Practical Guide to Better Breathing
- Living Better with ASTHMA: A Doctor's Practical Guide to Asthma Control
- SLEEP APNEA, INSOMNIA & OTHER SLEEP DISORDERS: A Doctor's Practical Guide to Better Sleep & Better Health
- Protect Your KIDNEYS: A Doctor's Practical Guide to Kidney Health & Prevention
- PROSTATE HEALTH After 40: A Doctor's Practical Guide to Early Detection & Care
- ARTHRITIS: A Doctor's Practical Guide to Pain Control & Mobility
- A Doctor's Practical Guide to Fixing BACK PAIN Step by Step
- A Doctor's Practical Guide to Understanding & Managing GOUT & URIC ACID and Preventing Complications
- COMMON SKIN & HAIR PROBLEMS: A Doctor's Practical Guide to Skin & Hair Care
- DEMENTIA & MEMORY LOSS: A Doctor's Practical Guide to Prevention & Management
- Doctor, Why Am I TIRED All the Time? Fixing Fatigue & Getting Your Energy Back

9 781971 672526

Printed by Libri Plureos GmbH in Hamburg, Germany